Anxiety Warrior

ELKE SCHOLZ

Ryan Brown, Yvonne Heath, Jill Hewlett,
Bari McFarland and Suzanne Witt-Foley

The
Artist's
Reply

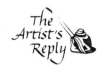

The
Artist's
Reply

Published by The Artist's Reply
Bracebridge, Ontario, Canada

ISBN 978-0-9736023-7-1 (pbk.)
ISBN 978-0-9736023-9-5 (epub)
ISBN 978-0-9736023-8-8 (mobi)

Cover art, design, typesetting:
Magdalene Carson, New Leaf Publication Design

Library and Archives Canada Cataloguing in Publication
Scholz, Elke, 1957-, author
Anxiety warrior / Elke Scholz ; [with contributions by] Ryan Brown,
Yvonne Heath, Jill Hewlett, Bari McFarland and Suzanne Witt-Foley.
Includes bibliographical references.
Issued in print and electronic formats.
ISBN 978-0-9736023-7-1 (softcover).
– ISBN 978-0-9736023-8-8 (Kindle).
– ISBN 978-0-9736023-9-5 (EPUB)
1. Anxiety. 2. Anxiety – Treatment. I. Title.
BF575.A6S36   2017   152.4'6   C2017-901990-2
C2017-901991-0

This book is written in Canadian English.

PERMISSIONS
Every attempt has been made to locate the sources of photographs
and other visuals. Should there be errors or omissions, please
contact the author for correction in future printings.

DISCLAIMER
The author and contributors of this book do not dispense medical
advice or prescribe the use of any technique as a form of treatment for
physical, emotional, mental or medical problems without the advice of
a physician, either directly or indirectly. The intent of the author and
contributors is to offer only general information in a general nature to
help you in your exploration for spiritual and emotional well-being.
In the event you use any of this information for yourself or others, the
author and contributors assume no responsibility for your actions.

To all of you,
there is an Anxiety Warrior within you.
We can do this!

Contents

Empowering Your Anxiety Warrior

Foreword

If I can sum up why I enjoy Elke's approach to psychotherapy so much, it would be the phrase *"Communicating with the body."* You will not only read this phrase in this book, but this theme is woven throughout the entirety of her approach and philosophy.

Our modern approach to health care has needed a revision for some time now, and here we have a fantastic example of that brave next step forward. I purposefully use the word *brave* for two reasons.

One is a nod to the prevailing model of fighting against a broken body/mind. Most of the approaches in health care are to fix a problem, dysfunction, or disorder. Our weak bodies, unbalanced hormones, and disrupted brain chemistry are due to some genetic fault, and it is up to the medical establishment to fix and/or support us through this. We need to fight, overcome, battle, and follow the mantra of mind over matter, or more accurately, medicine over mind and matter.

Just reading these last few sentences, I would ask you to check into how you are feeling. Somewhat disempowered and depressed? Hardly a good way to initiate the healing process.

My second reason for using *brave* is to acknowledge the real bravery in picking up a book such as this one and embarking on a fruitful journey towards wholeness. Yes, it will require some effort, introspection, and responsibility (the best things in life often do). However, the reward, in addition to providing tools and a plan to ease your anxiety, is to rediscover your friend that is your body.

I cannot think of a better teacher than our bodies, and I cannot think of a better instructor than Elke, who will unlock the codes, clues, and signals that our bodies use to communicate to us.

If you have ever had the honour of attending one of Elke's workshops, then you are already aware of the value of this book. Personally

I have attended a number of her workshops dealing with anxiety and the brain, and found them not only informative, but life-changing. Elke is both knowledgeable and down-to-earth practical, and I was very pleased to learn of her intent to compile her list of resources into this book. You will learn how anxiety manifests, where it originates, as well as vital information to help you understand how your brain works. In short, this book aims to explain and clarify why you feel what you do, and offers you ways to manage your anxiety so that you can live a productive, happy life.

Elke's approach encompasses both *simplicity* and *complexity*. The workings of the brain and the condition of anxiety are complex, and Elke's knowledge of this is at a high level. She is able to both understand and speak the lingo of neurology, and brings the latest findings into her practice and treatment strategies. At the same time, she is able to make simple use of this knowledge. You will learn and you will know what to do with that knowledge.

I acknowledge and appreciate your decision to help yourself. Even to pick this book up and pause to read this foreword is a significant step. You have made a good choice, and I anticipate that you will use this resource again and again. In closing, I suggest that you touch your body right now, even just your arm, and know that soon you will be working with this body towards a better life and a better future. And if you have the good fortune to attend one of Elke's workshops, be sure to bring a friend — they will benefit too!

Dr. Nick Bianchi

Dr. Nick Bianchi, B.SC. (KIN), D.C., is a chiropractor, published author, and speaker practicing in Bracebridge, Ontario. His model of health care and his clinical approach include a whole-person wellness perspective and patient education. Elke is a favourite guest speaker of his patients and of Dr. Nick as well.

Acknowledgements

First, I would like to thank my children, Alec and Emma. They may not always understand me and my anxiety, however, they love me all the same. They are my most important achievement. Writing a book on anxiety has itself been a source of anxiety for me, and we have found some humour in that!

Thank you to my mom, Gisela. She may not have ever named it in me, though she knew my migraines and flu symptoms as a child were real for me.

Thank you to my dad, Peter, for his example of believing that there is a better way, and for his determination. He was the letter writer, he was the risk taker, and believed in his dreams. At the age of 24, he moved his young family to Canada.

I thank author Lucinda Bassett for her work. In reading her book *Panic to Power* for a friend I finally recognized my own anxiety. And I thank my good family doctor, Dr. Allison Small, who took the time to get to know me. She waited and she trusted me to come to her when I needed to, for she saw the anxiety in me before I saw it myself.

To my dear colleagues and professionals who inspire me, I am grateful for the network of mutual support and encouragement we have created. While we may not see each other often, we are always available and in touch, which is sustaining and motivating.

I am also grateful to my friends and community for all their assistance, sponsorship, encouragement and enthusiasm in the book and The Anxiety Warrior Project: Celebrating Living Life Well, a symposium held in April 2017, and where this book was officially launched. Both the book and the project have been a collective effort and certainly not a solitary journey.

Thank you Susanne Mika, my assistant, for believing in me and the work.

xiv *Acknowledgements*

To Magdalene Carson, for listening and chatting with me, not
always about designing, for letting me cry and laugh. For all the col-
laborative fun we have when we are on fire about designing! Exalted
warrior!

Thank you, Ted Lute for fresh eyes, at the final hour for a read and
critique. You are an avid reader and happily said 'yes'!

Thank you to all the contributors. You are so passionate about
your work and about empowering people.

And to all of you around the world, who believe in me and the
work. People have asked me where I get the energy. Your letters,
emails, personal stories and triumphs go right to my heart and fuel
my fire.

Introduction

Are you reading this book because anxiety has become a constant companion? Is it with you everywhere, all the time? Or hits you unexpectedly? Does it feel like the worst feeling ever? Do you feel like a victim losing? Or like an empowered warrior? When you feel anxiety, it feels like you are fighting it. Yet somehow anxiety can be a gift, an opportunity. A battle that does not have violent casualities; however, the casualities are the layers of causes that alert us to anxiety. The battle then is to overcome and to manage these causes.

In the following pages I share what I have learned from years of research and practice about managing anxiety. I also introduce you to brilliant contributors — writers, speakers, teachers, and facilitators who offer unique insights and perspectives. They are passionate about their topics and live them. By applying the thoughts, ideas, and strategies in this book that resonate with you, you will be able to better manage your anxiety, and enjoy more fully all the good things in your life.

I know from my own personal, and professional experience that we *can* lower our levels of anxiety.

Today I manage my anxiety.

I have had anxiety all my life, but I did not always know it. As a child I had migraines, tummy aches, and flu-ish feelings, so often that I had to miss school. My mom believed me, however; my dad did not think that I was truly sick. Often I would be sick before a test or presentation. I also would cry easily in class if teachers raised their voice, even when it was not directed at me. I remember as a teen feeling angry, hopeless, misunderstood, and very alone, until I met two very special teachers, Mrs. Yeo, my Creative English teacher, and Mr. Hodwitz, my Drama teacher. They saved my life. After their classes I felt I could be okay in the world.

In my 20s at times I would feel 'out of myself'. At the time, I could not recall how or why it came on. An urgent feeling would hijack me and I felt a need to run away, usually to a nearby meadow. I felt I had to hide. Usually, I would run along the beach and curl up in a fetal position beside a dune until the feeling subsided and I felt safe and could breathe normally again. At that time I thought I was 'crazy'. It was my secret. As I write here, it is the first time I have ever told anyone this. I know now that it was trauma and anxiety related. That is another story.

Twenty years ago I went through periods when I had trouble getting out of bed. I would send my son off to school and then go back to bed until he came home. Sometimes I would get dressed, sometimes not. When out of bed, I would sit and stare at my work or sit outside and stare. I had no idea that I might be anxious or depressed. I felt immobilized and had no idea about how to get out and be different. I denigrated myself. I had gone to see one counsellor and she said I was 'my own worst enemy'. I really did not know what she meant by that, and I was too vulnerable to risk asking. That comment only made me feel worse. Looking back, I see that she did not give me strategies or direction so that I could learn how to be my own best friend.

Fifteen years ago, I didn't sleep for two years. I would not fight it and instead lay awake and rested as best I could so I could work and carry on. Friends encouraged me to go to the doctor because I could get very sick. I decided to go for a spa weekend of Turkish sauna, hot tub, and massage. My body was exhausted, I could barely walk and get ready for bed, yet I stared awake at the ceiling all night. I knew then that I needed to see my doctor. In tears I told her that I could not sleep and wondered if I had anxiety? She said yes, and that she had been waiting for me to come to her so I could hear her.

My good doctor would not give me sleeping pills unless I promised her that I would go to therapy. I was affronted, as I didn't think that I needed therapy. However, I agreed since I needed so badly to sleep. This began a journey of discovery that shaped my personal and professional life.

I do remember some key points of change and awareness.

Twenty years ago, I remember driving my silver Ford station wagon to a workshop. It was a fine sunny day, traffic was good and I felt good. About 20 minutes later I felt sad and my mood dropped. I felt sick. Nothing had changed except that I was further down the highway. I noticed this, changed channels in my mind and thought of a fun happy fantasy. At the time I did not fully realize what I had done.

Twelve years ago, I remember very clearly driving in my van down Manitoba Street in Bracebridge, on another sunny day, thinking *I have all my fingers and toes, I can see, hear, I have a lovely home, I am able, healthy, and have two great kids, so why am I not dancing in the streets celebrating?* Instead, I felt horrible. I was determined to change.

Have you ever met those people who, when you ask how they are, say "SUPER! GREAT!" And they mean it. I wanted to be one of those people.

I was determined to change channels. And so, I began this journey of discovery.

I'm sharing my personal and professional experiences with you because every week half a million Canadians will miss work due to stress/anxiety.[1] About 30% of girls and 20% of boys have had an anxiety disorder, according to data from the U.S. National Institute of Mental Health,[2] and most people who come to my private clinic suffer from anxiety. The success that my clients have achieved and the positive response to my talks on anxiety have fuelled my passion about lowering levels of anxiety in an approachable way and making it easy and accessible for everyone who needs it.

Can you imagine a life without anxiety? Is it reasonable to think one could not ever have anxiety again? That is not likely. Anxiety is part of the human spectrum of feelings. Anxiety can be a gift or a clue, notifying us that we need to pay attention to something, that perhaps something is amiss. However, we can have a life where anxiety does not control our lives, our decisions, and our choices.

When I wake up with anxiety, I go through a mental checklist (more about the checklist on page 37). Within 10 to 30 minutes, the anxiety is usually gone. This is just one of the ways in which I have learned that a life managing anxiety is attainable.

What does a life managing anxiety feel like?

It feels empowering. It feels like I have a choice. It feels like I can. It feels like I have a right to be happy. It feels like I am able. And it feels like I am worthy of thriving.

Now imagine a life in which you're telling people you feel "GREAT," and you mean it!

Notes

1. Insurance Journal 2003, as cited by the Government of Canada in *The Human Face of Mental Health and Mental Illness in Canada,* 2006, pg. 41.
2. Cited in "Teen Depression and Anxiety: Why the Kids Are Not Alright," an article by Susanna Schrobsdorff for *Time Magazine,* posted October 27, 2016; http://time.com/4547322/american-teens-anxious-depressed-overwhelmed/.

What Is Anxiety?

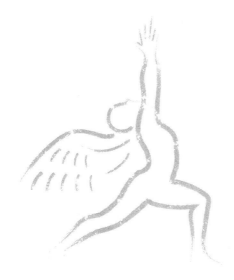

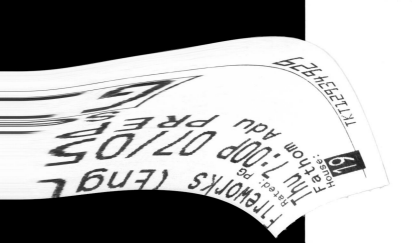

What Is Anxiety?

I wonder if anxiety is worse than it was 20 to 40 years ago, or if we have been conditioned to be positive, happy people and fail if we feel otherwise? Or perhaps we are anxious every day and get worn out and overwhelmed. Or perhaps we are set up to be anxious through media and social messages.

Studies suggest that our anxiety level is generally higher than it was 30 years ago, and it's starting earlier in our lives. The proportion of 15- to 16-year-olds reporting that they frequently feel anxious or depressed has doubled in the last 30 years, for boys from 1 in 30 to 2 in 30, and for girls from 1 in 10 to 2 in 10.[1]

A *useful check-in scale.*

I would like to introduce a useful check-in scale. I find it is helpful for both myself and clients to have a scale to check in, 0 to 10. By giving your anxiety a number, sometimes it is easier to identify. Zero is no disturbance, so at 0 you are calm, settled, and relaxed. As the anxiety level grows, the numbers get higher.

For example, I might feel a little jittery or nervous, maybe even excited, and that might be a 2 or 3, and is very manageable. However, I know when I reach a 4, I want to begin my strategies. I do not want to go higher, because then the numbers escalate quickly for me.

I know that my 10 means heart pain, laboured breathing, nausea, and so on. It is hard to come down from a 10: my thoughts do not go together and it feels like circuitry misfiring. So when I notice that I am at a 4, I begin my strategies.

Some people are fine at a 5 or 6. It is important to know your limits.

It does not does not matter if your 2 is different from my 2. What is important is that the scale works for you and you understand what the numbers and levels mean for you.

At the beginning of this book, perhaps even after reading the definitions, you may want to check in and give yourself a number from 0 to 10.

Also check in when you wake in the mornings: Where are you at? What number would you give yourself?

Try a creative practice and then check in again. Using the scale will help you create your supports and resources. It will be a barometer for your anxiety and will give you clues as to what exercises are most useful for you.

Children who understand numbers from 0 to 10 quickly grasp this scale and can give their parents feedback on how they are feeling.

Appearing below are definitions of various terms related to anxiety. Further on, I'll tell you about seven types of anxiety. Understanding the various forms and layers of anxiety is the first step in managing it.

Anxiety: Feelings of worry, nervousness, or unease, typically about an imminent event or an uncertain outcome. Feelings of concern, apprehension, unease, fearfulness, disquiet, agitation, angst, tension, twitchiness, nervousness. Mostly felt in anticipation of something happening.

Pathological anxiety, psychiatric meaning: A nervous disorder characterized by a state of excessive uneasiness and apprehension, typically with compulsive behaviour or panic attacks. When anxiety is a problem it affects our health, our well-being, and our happiness. When anxiety stops us from doing something, like going out of the house, going shopping, driving, taking a course, going to a party, or visiting family, it is a problem.

Worry: From an old English word 'wrygan', meaning 'to strangle'. Allowing your mind to dwell on difficulties or troubles, fretting, being concerned, agonizing, overthinking, brooding, panicking, getting worked up, getting stressed, getting in a state, stewing, or tormenting oneself. Worry tends to be repetitive.

Fear versus anxiety: Fear is something you feel when you are threatened, while anxiety is being afraid in anticipation of something happening. They both have the same physiological response in the body. Fear is when you are in the woods and a bear is coming after you. You are afraid, you must make a decision; you must run or take cover. Fear is an important emotion

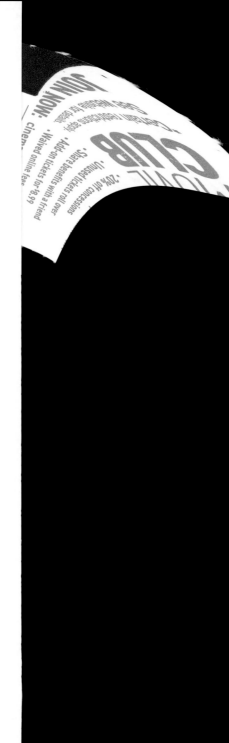

that has kept the human species alive. Anxiety is when you *anticipate* that a bear may come after you.

Chronic worry: Have you ever had thoughts that keep looping as they if they were on a reel, returning over and over again? Chronic worry is repetitive.

Anxiety can manifest in many ways, such as butterflies in the stomach, tightly curled toes, shaking, stiff neck, sore back, indigestion, fidgeting, picking, nail biting, hair pulling, restlessness, increased heart rate, sweating, flushed cheeks, rash, hives, nausea, stomach ache, headaches, migraines, weight loss, weight gain, tension, stress, fatigue, exhaustion, restlessness, busy mind, looping thoughts, adrenalin, Obsessive Compulsive Disorder (OCD), insomnia, agitation, clenched teeth, teeth grinding, locked jaw, Irritable Bowel Syndrome (IBS), chest pains, shortness of breath, lack of concentration, lack of patience, anger, and more.

Anxiety has many different layers and degrees of intensity. The more aware you are of these layers, the greater your ability to change them or manage them. Know your limits. One of my participants uses her anxiety to motivate and energize herself. For me, my anxiety is a clue that something is going on that I need to take care of. So I use a mental checklist to explore its possible cause. You can find my personal mental checklist at the beginning of the next section, *Empowering Your Anxiety Warrior*.

I invite you to keep in mind how any of these signals may be useful and/or an opportunity. What is anxiety telling you? What is its signal to you?

The warrior becomes self-assured, self-confident, assertive, and positive.

Depression

The Mayo Clinic defines depression as a mood disorder that causes a persistent feeling of sadness and loss of interest. Also called major depressive disorder or clinical depression, it affects how you feel, think, and behave, and can lead to a variety of emotional and physical problems.[2]

A mood disorder is a general emotional state or mood that is distorted or inconsistent with your circumstances. Here's an example: At different times in our lives we may suffer from grief and sadness.

People with mood disorders suffer for much longer periods of time. They feel as if they cannot control their mood or emotions. If it's possible that you or someone you know is suffering from a mood disorder, consider seeking a professional assessment.

Depression and anxiety often occur together. If you are suffering from one, you are likely suffering from both. Sometimes anxiety occurs as a symptom of depression and vice versa.

We hear about depression in many different ways. It is part of being human; feeling sad or depressed happens to all of us. After a visit or an exciting weekend and the house is quiet again, you might feel depressed, though you may call it 'low'. Sometimes we might feel 'blue' or 'low' for a short time and it lifts without intervention. Feeling depressed for two weeks or more, with the loss of interest or enjoyment of any activities, may be a major depressive episode. People can recover from major depression but also experience it again. People rarely seek help for this, and even when they do it is not often identified.

Depression affects a person's productivity. People miss work and cannot work as effectively.

Here are some outward signs of depression:

+ Looking sad, dejected or anxious, or speaking in a monotone.

+ Having decreased energy, feeling tired, having slowed thinking, and feeling restless. (Some people describe themselves as feeling numb and beyond tears.)

+ Crying and withdrawal.

+ Loss of interest in personal hygiene and appearance.

+ A lack of motivation in daily activities.

Depressed people have a negative world view; they think negatively of themselves and the future. They feel hopeless and helpless. They see events around them as evidence of personal flaws. They hold a sense of worthlessness and guilt. They say things like, "I can't do anything right," "No one loves me," "Things will always be rough," and "Life is not worth living." They feel sad, anxious, guilty, angry, impatient, and unworthy.

Thoughts are affected, due to regular self-criticism, worry, negative outlook, and difficultly focusing and in making decisions. We might feel confused and think about death and suicide.

Physically, depressed people might feel tired or exhausted. They might eat too much or too little. They may want to sleep all the time or have insomnia. They may lose their sexual drive. Sometimes they have inexplicable aches and pains.

There are different levels of depression and not everyone will have all the symptoms at the same time. Again, if you are concerned, seek a professional opinion.

When anxiety disrupts your life, it's a problem.

Not all types of anxiety qualify as an anxiety disorder. It may feel very uncomfortable, unbearable, and, when unmanageable, very depressing.

If you feel your anxiety is causing a problem in your life, it may be beneficial to seek help. Some anxiety in life is normal. However, anxiety that disrupts your quality of life is problematic when it stops you from doing things you love, accepting that job you want, or fulfilling a dream you have.

Even though different categories of anxiety have names, anxiety can be layered. Don't worry where you may fit among the categories. If your anxiety is stopping you from doing something, seek professional help.

No matter what type of anxiety you're dealing with, anxiety can be managed by the following strategies:

+ Explore and understand the possibility of a specific type of anxiety.

+ Accept your anxiety as a gift, a signal, an opportunity, a message.

+ Identify and understand the causes and triggers for your anxiety.

+ Use the scale 0 to 10 to identify the intensity of your anxiety.

+ Know your limits, (sleep, hunger, amount, and type of stressors).

✦ Perhaps break down your anxiety into smaller layers.

✦ Manage the easy layers first, right away.

✦ Change your lifestyle to lower the anxiety.

✦ Practice your strategies.

✦ Create your own daily routine and practice it daily, especially when you feel pleasant.

If I could only give you two words from this book, they would be 'awareness' and 'practice'. Become aware so you know what to change/ modify/manage and practice your strategies. Life is a process and a practice for all of us!

Below, we'll examine seven types of anxiety. More than one may apply at the same time, or at different times in your life depending on the situation.

1. Generalized Anxiety Disorder (GAD)

Generalized Anxiety Disorder (GAD), is the most common and widespread type of anxiety. GAD affects tens of millions of people throughout the world.

GAD is best described as an ongoing state of mental and/or physical tension and nervousness, either without a clear cause or without a break from the anxiety.

If you feel yourself constantly on edge, worried, anxious, or stressed (either physically or mentally) and it's disrupting your life, you may have Generalized Anxiety Disorder. Remember, some anxiety is a natural part of life, and it's normal to feel some degree of occasional anxiety. However, when that anxiety appears to occur for no reason or is out of proportion to the cause, you may have Generalized Anxiety Disorder.

The following are the most common symptoms associated with GAD:

✦ Constant restlessness, irritation, edginess, or a feeling of being without control.

✦ Fatigue, lethargy, or generally low energy levels (feeling exhausted or drained).

✦ Tense muscles, especially on the back, neck, and shoulders.

✦ Difficulty concentrating or focusing on tasks and/or activities.

✦ Negative thoughts — 'disaster thinking'.

When the mental and/or physical anxieties are persistent and don't go away, it may be GAD.

Generalized Anxiety Disorder can be very common in those struggling with other anxiety disorders, such as panic disorder and Obsessive Compulsive Disorder.

2. Social phobia

Some people suffer from 'social phobia', or fear of social situations. Some degree of social phobia is normal. Small degrees of shyness in public places, or discomfort while public speaking, are natural in most people and do not imply an anxiety problem.

However, when that fear keeps you away from social settings, you may be suffering from social phobia. Social phobia occurs when the shyness is intense and the idea of socializing or speaking with the public, strangers, authority figures, or possibly even your friends causes you noticeable anxiety and fear.

If you have social phobia, public situations feel particularly painful and distressing. There can be a constant fear of being judged, observed, remarked upon, or avoided. Those with social phobia also often have an irrational fear of doing something stupid or embarrassing.

What makes this more than just shyness is that those fears cause you to avoid healthy socializing situations altogether. Those with social phobia often experience one or more of the following issues:

✦ Feeling hopeless or fearful with unfamiliar people or in unfamiliar situations.

✦ Obsession over being watched, observed, or judged, whether by strangers or friends.

✦ Feeling overwhelming anxiety in any social situation.

✦ Severe fear of public speaking, beyond what one would consider 'normal'.

✦ Anxiety about the idea of social situations, even when not in one.

✦ Intense issues about meeting new people or speaking up when you need to speak.

Many people with social phobia avoid any and all social situations as best they can, so as to avoid the discomfort of anxiety.

3. Panic disorder

Panic disorder is a debilitating anxiety disorder that is different from GAD. Panic disorder is not about 'panicking' in a given situation.

For example, panicking about being attacked by a bear is natural. Panic *disorder* is when you experience severe feelings of doom that cause both mental and physical symptoms so intense that some people become hospitalized, believing that something is dangerously wrong with their health.

Panic disorder is characterized by:

1. Panic attacks. These are intense physical and mental sensations that may be triggered by stress, anxiety, or by nothing at all. They often involve mental distress, but are best recognized by their physical symptoms, including:

✦ Rapid heartbeat (heart palpitations or irregular/fast-paced heart rhythms).

✦ Excessive sweating or hot/cold flashes.

✦ Tingling sensations, numbness, or weakness in the body.

✦ Depersonalization (feeling like you're outside yourself)

✦ Difficulty breathing or feeling as though you've taken a deep breath.

✦ Light-headedness or dizziness.

✦ Chest pain or stomach ache.

✦ Digestive problems and/or discomfort.

2. Fear of getting panic attacks. This may have some or all of the above physical symptoms, and may also involve seemingly unrelated symptoms, such as headaches, ear pressure, and more. All of these symptoms feel very real, which is why those who experience this fear often seek medical attention.

Panic attacks of both types are also known for their mental 'symptoms', which peak about 10 minutes into an attack. These include:

✦ A feeling of doom, or the feeling as though you're about to die.

✦ A feeling of helplessness, or feeling like you're no longer yourself.

Contrary to popular belief, it's possible for the physical symptoms of panic attacks to come before *or* after anxiety, meaning that you can experience physical symptoms before experiencing, say, the fear of death. That is why many people may not associate their symptoms with anxiety, and instead associate them with the possibility of physical health problems.

Panic disorder can be very hard to control without help. Seeking assistance for your panic attacks is an important tool for stopping them, so that you can learn the techniques necessary to master panic.

You can also have panic disorder without experiencing many panic attacks. If you live in constant fear of a panic attack, you may also qualify for a panic disorder diagnosis. In such cases, your anxiety may resemble Generalized Anxiety Disorder, with the difference that the fear in this case is known.

4. Agoraphobia

Agoraphobia is more common in adults. Agoraphobia is the fear of going out in public, open spaces, or being in unfamiliar places. Many people who suffer from agoraphobia rarely leave their homes. Some can travel from home to work. Some can go to the grocery store or other familiar places but experience intense, debilitating fear anywhere else.

I had a client, a young man who was able to go to work. He was very responsible and reliable. He could go for drives in his own vehicle. He even could drive for his employer, as long as he had minimal contact with other people. His worry was that he might have a panic attack while shopping or being in any public place where people might notice that he was nervous. So he stayed home.

Many people who have agoraphobia also have panic disorder. People experience panic attacks in public places, so they start to avoid more and more places in order to avoid panic attacks.

Some people experience agoraphobia after traumatic events. They fear losing control psychologically and physically, which causes them to avoid social situations.

There are different types of agoraphobia:

+ Obsessive fear of socializing with groups of people, regardless of whether or not you know them.

+ Severe stress or anxiety whenever you're in an environment other than your home, or an environment where you're not in control.

+ Feelings of tension and stress during regular activities, such as going to the store, talking with strangers, or even just stepping outdoors.

+ Preoccupation with how to protect yourself or find safety in the event that a crisis occurs, whether there is cause for concern or not.

+ Your own fears are keeping you hostage, stopping you from going out, and living life.

Many people experience moments where they feel vulnerable outdoors and prefer to stay safe in their homes. However, when the fear seems to continue for a long period of time, or is holding you back from living an enjoyable life, you may have agoraphobia.

5. Phobias

Phobias are intense fears of objects, scenarios, animals, etc. Phobias generally bring about disaster thinking (believing the worst will happen) or avoidance behaviours (doing whatever it takes to avoid the phobia).

An example of a common phobia is arachnophobia, or fear of spiders. Very few spiders are likely to bite and even fewer are dangerous, yet many people experience a feeling of severe dread at the sight of a spider. Other examples of phobias involve snakes, mice, airplanes, thunderstorms, clowns, blood, and so on.

Phobias are considered an anxiety disorder, even though some people can go their entire lives with a phobia and not require treatment. For example, if you have a fear of chickens but live nowhere near a farm, it is not a problem for you.

Alternatively, you may experience severe 'what if' scenarios everywhere you go, including disaster thinking or feeling helpless/hopeless in public situations.

If at any point your life starts to change as a result of your phobia, then you may have a real problem. Phobias commonly cause:

+ Excessive and/or continuous fear of a specific thing, situation or event.

+ Instant feelings of terror when confronted with the subject of the phobia.

+ Inability to control the fear.

+ Going to great lengths to avoid the situation or object that causes the fear.

+ Changing and limiting life routines because of the fear.

For some people with severe phobias, the mere idea of the object they fear (even if it is not present) causes stress or anxiety, or otherwise affects their life.

Many people have small phobias they can manage, but if a phobia ever starts to genuinely affect your ability to live your life, you may need to seek professional help.

6. Post Traumatic Stress Disorder (PTSD)

PTSD is an anxiety disorder that can develop after one or many traumatic events. It can also happen over a period of time, and/or be a collection of what we call 'small t's' and/or 'big T's' in Eye Movement

Desensitization and Reprocessing (EMDR; see the *Glossary*, page 154, for the full meaning).

PTSD affects people both psychologically and physically. In most cases, the person with PTSD is the one who experienced the traumatic event, though it's possible to get PTSD by simply witnessing an event or injury, or even by discovering that someone close to you dealt with a traumatic event. Therapists can get secondary trauma from hearing traumatic stories.

People with PTSD may avoid behaviours, events, things, and even other people who may remind them of the trauma. Many people with PTSD also experience issues with their emotional thinking and future. Some feel a disinterest in or detachment from love. Others become emotionally numb. Some feel that a dark cloud follows them. Others become convinced they're destined to die. Any and all of these emotional struggles may be common in people with PTSD.

Symptoms of PTSD include:

✦ flashbacks, the most well-known symptom of PTSD. Those with PTSD often relive the trauma mentally and physically, as though it is happening again. Flashbacks come as intrusive thoughts, or nightmares, and/or night terrors, whether triggered or not.

✦ triggers, which are often related to the event, such as smells, sounds, tastes, feelings, colours, and so on. A trigger can revive the memory.

✦ anxiety and/or hypervigilance over recurrence. As with panic attacks, you may have PTSD if you experience:

  ✧ Regular, daily anxiety over the idea of a repeat event.

  ✧ Hypervigilance about certain locations and events, such as swimming pools, driving, fires, and so on.

Post-traumatic stress depletes your resources and resilience. You may be short tempered, less patient, and anger easily. Perhaps you may be startled or frighten easily, and/or have trouble sleeping.

If you suspect that you have PTSD, get outside help. PTSD can affect people for years after the event occurs, possibly even the rest of their lives.

7. Obsessive Compulsive Disorder (OCD)

Compulsions and obsessions are similar, but present themselves in different ways:

- ✦ *Obsessions*, which are thought based. They're a preoccupation with a specific thought, usually negative or fearful, that a person cannot get rid of no matter how hard they try.

- ✦ *Compulsions*, which are behaviour based. They're a 'need' to perform an action or activity, often in a very specific way: as hard as the person tries, they can't stop themselves from performing the behaviour.

Those with OCD often exhibit behaviours and fears that are not only confusing to people around them, but which may also be confusing to the person with OCD.

For example, an obsession would be worrying that your friend will tire of you, while a compulsion would be feeling anxious if you do not touch a doorknob before you leave the house. In many cases, the feelings are linked: those with OCD may feel that they need to touch a doorknob, or their friends may tire of them.

You can have compulsions without obsessions, though in most cases sufferers will experience severe stress if they do not respond to the urge of the compulsion. You can also have obsessions without compulsions (such as the fear of germs), but in many cases these fears will lead to a compulsion, such as having to wash your hands over and over again.

Obsessive Thought Patterns

Many people with OCD go through a variety of thought processes that lead to their obsessions and compulsions. The following are a few examples of obsessive thought patterns and compulsive behaviour patterns.

- ✦ You find yourself 'obsessed' with things that you appear to be the only one worrying about.

- ✦ You try to shake away those thoughts when they occur, usually by performing an action.

✦ You find that the action doesn't work, and ultimately the obsession continues.

✦ You find yourself upset over being unable to shake the thoughts.

✦ You find that the worse you feel, the more you seem to obsess over those thoughts.

Compulsive behaviour patterns

✦ You experience anxiety, often over an obsession (although not necessarily).

✦ You perform an action that appears to reduce that anxiety slightly.

✦ You turn to this action to relieve your anxiety, until it becomes a ritual.

✦ You find that you absolutely have to perform this behaviour, or your anxiety becomes overwhelming.

✦ You repeat the action and reinforce the behaviour.

Compulsions and obsessions may appear to be very unusual, and it's possible to know that they're irrational and/or strange, but people with OCD still feel they can't control them.

There are many types of anxiety. People may experience them together, or separately in varying intensities. The next chapter discusses the many layers of anxiety.

Notes

1 These findings are from the Nuffield Foundation's Changing Adolescence Programme and are published by Policy Press in *Changing Adolescence: Social trends and mental health* (http://policypress.co.uk/changing-adolescence), which explores how social change has affected young people's behaviour, mental health and transitions toward adulthood.
2 The Mayo Clinic is an internationally recognized nonprofit organization committed to clinical practice, education, and research, providing expert, whole-person care to everyone who needs healing. www.mayoclinic.org

Eleven Layers of Anxiety

Over the years, I have discovered that anxiety has many layers that may build up over time and which can gradually or quickly prevent us from enjoying our lives. In the previous chapter we discussed various types of anxiety. In this chapter I describe eleven of these layers — contributing factors that may intensify the type(s) of anxiety we feel.

I have also discovered, along with my clients, that examining and addressing these layers can lower the intensity of our anxiety and lower the scale. Some are easy to address. Others may require time and effort.

We can usually tolerate different stresses at the same time. However, we all have a threshold. If there are too many and we exceed our personal limit, we can quickly get into a highly anxious state. Your own experience and trial and error will show you what your limits are. As you build your skills and resilience, you will likely recover more quickly from anxiety.

The first step is to understand which layers are contributing to your particular anxiety. Elsewhere in this book we'll talk about ways of dealing with the anxiety.

1. Substances

Substances such as caffeine, sugar, alcohol, and drugs, whether pharmaceutical or recreational, can affect the brain and cause anxiety symptoms. Nicotine is known to stimulate the body and makes the heart work harder. Smokers will say that a smoke calms them. However, smokers tend to be more anxious and do not sleep as well as non-smokers. Excessive salt can stress the body. Too much salt can deplete the body of potassium, which is important in the functioning of the nervous system. It also raises blood pressure, putting a strain on the heart and arteries. Simple starches can quickly turn into sugar in the body. If you are sensitive to sugars, your body may react with restlessness, palpitations, and anxiety.

Edmund J. Bourne states in his books that there are about 5,000 chemical additives used in commercial food processing. Little is known about the long-term effects of these chemicals. Some have been known to create adverse reactions:

> *Case study:* I have a sensitivity to sugars, and at suppertime if I have pasta made with bleached white flour, I am up all night. I also have a cut-off time for chocolate and caffeine: if I have these by 2:00 p.m., my body can metabolize them. It takes my body 5 to 6 hours to metabolize the sugars. On the other hand, my brother and my mom can have coffee just before bedtime and fall asleep.

It is important to know your body and your limits.

If the brain does not have enough water, it can send signals to the body that are similar to anxiety.

Alcohol depletes the body of fluid and can induce reactions similar to anxiety. Wine and alcohol contain a lot of sugar. Decaffeinated products and green tea still have caffeine in them.

> *Case study:* A client called me, quite agitated and upset. She feared an upcoming panic attack. I asked her if anything unusual was going on in her life, and she said no. I asked how often she felt like this, and she answered, "Pretty much every day." Then I asked what she'd eaten that day. She said she felt too sick to eat. She'd had a cup of coffee first thing in the morning and then felt nauseous, so she did not eat. However, she then had about seven more cups of coffee. She also relayed that she had not been sleeping well. I suggested that she wean herself off coffee and call me in a week's time. When we connected again, she said she felt tremendously different. Her anxiety levels were lower and she was sleeping much better.

Again, know your limits.

Other food sensitivities can cause anxiety. If you suspect food sensitivities, you can get extensive blood work done to check. Ask your family doctor. You can also get food testing done through laboratories and naturopathic doctors. In my private practice, many of my clients have discovered food sensitivities. Once they have modified their diets, their moods become much improved. I talk more about this in the *Strategies* section (page 66).

Deficiencies of Vitamins B1, B2, B6, and B12 can lead to anxiety and restlessness. If you are concerned about supplement care and Vitamin deficiencies, consult your health practitioner.

2. Physiological

Physiological conditions can mimic, trigger, or intensify anxiety. Being active is a way for many people to manage their anxiety levels. Our bodies produce endorphins (the feel-good hormones) when we are physically active, which helps to alleviate anxious feelings.

Hormone imbalance and/or thyroid imbalance can generate symptoms similar to anxiety. Being low on iron will also generate symptoms of depression and anxiety. If you are experiencing anxiety and still don't know why after reading this chapter, then ask your family doctor to run some tests to help identify possible causes. In my therapy practice, I usually ask, "What are you eating? What do you do for activities? How are you sleeping? If you are not sleeping well, is insomnia the cause or a result of anxiety, or both?" Lack of sleep can also cause anxiety-like symptoms. In this case, medical and/or mental health professional advice may be useful.

3. Reality

Is there something real that needs attending to, such as a pending decision, multiple decisions, finding a job, managing finances, visiting someone? Looming deadlines for projects? Upcoming performances or presentations? Exams? Moving? Interviews? Court hearings? Conversations with professionals? Doctor's appointments? Surgery? Separation?

Here, fear, and anxiety can be useful indicators of very real issues we need to deal with. For example, are you worried about money? About paying bills? This may mean it's time to attend to your finances. Check out your bank account. Consider budgeting, perhaps debt consolidation, and/or a debt reduction program. It may mean research, and working with a financial coach. It is amazing the resources we have in our society to help with finances. I once attended a talk given by a colleague, who encouraged participants to let her provide them with a complementary session so that she could assess their finances and help them with planning. She suggested that people should do this even if they have no money to invest. She helps with planning for the future as well.

I took my friend up on her offer. I felt very vulnerable and generally embarrassed about the state of my finances. However, she had a way of making me feel comfortable, and once I got over my initial nervousness I felt better.

Case study: Sheila came into my private practice hysterical and weepy about her recent separation. She had trouble thinking and was blaming her past on her 'over-the-top anxiety'. She also believed others when they told her she was over the top. The truth was that she was currently living in her estranged husband's house with their two young daughters. Sheila had no private space and did not know when her ex-husband was coming or going. He did not respect her space. Her mother's support fell through when she could not secure a down payment for her on a house. Renting would trap her, adding to the time required to save for a reliable home for her and her two young children. At a 'Maslow hierarchy level' (see the *Glossary*, page 155) she was being challenged. She did not know where to live and how to survive. When I acknowledged her feelings and explained what may be causing her anxiety, she drew a large breath and her anxiety lowered enough for her to think more clearly.

Case study: A few years back I bought a house and studio on six acres in the country. Moving from a bungalow in town was a shock. Many challenges lay ahead of me, and every day for two years I woke up feeling nauseous and panicky. I had trouble thinking, I was so distraught. A local real-estate firm that was managing the sale caused me undue hardships, and the original owner had not disclosed the house's many weaknesses. One winter later, I realized that my house did not feel safe, it was cold in the winter and the hydro was costing me $12,000 a year (an increase of $9,000 from my bungalow.) The roof leaked in seven places. At the studio, the pipes kept freezing. Ants were eating my home. I had little money to fix the problems. Even though I was trying to build a private practice, I realized I needed to get my finances in order and make my house safe, so that I could feel safe. I needed to make this a priority, as it was affecting my health and my personal and professional lives.

I was able to re-mortgage the house and install a new roof; I fixed the windows, resolved the hydro issue, and installed a wood stove. I finally felt safe and cozy and calm.

Perhaps you feel nervous about seeing a doctor or having tests done. It is natural to feel some nervousness. Can you accept that some situations will make you feel nervous? You may have a sleepless night or two. This is natural. Can you be kind and gentle with yourself, know that this is natural and do some self-care?

How can you nurture yourself in a difficult situation and know that it will pass? Again, be aware of your limits and notice any other sources of anxiety.

4. Overstimulation

Cell phones, texting, computers, TV, gaming, all within reason are useful. However, when we exceed our limits, the stimulation is overwhelming, causing anxiety. In this world of rapid technology, we come to expect quick responses and messages. FOMO, 'fear-of-missing-out', has become a term for our fast-paced technical culture.

> *Case study:* Bonnie, a 17-year-old client, was having trouble sleeping. She reported getting 10 to 20 texts before bedtime from various friends. She was so conscientious that she felt she had to answer them all before going to bed. Of course this took long into the night. She was concerned about peer pressure and did not want to hurt anyone. Finally, she told her friends that she was shutting off her phone at 9:00 p.m. so she could do her homework and go to bed. She reported sleeping better and feeling better. When asked, Bonnie relayed that her friends accepted her turning her phone off.

Some people watch TV or the computer before bedtime. Many studies show that the blue screen tricks the brain into thinking that it is daytime, so that it does not want to shut off. Take a break from any screen for an hour or two to let your brain settle down so you can sleep.

I could follow this advice too. Many times I am inspired to write at night, and then I cannot fall asleep for a few hours.

5. Cultural and social beliefs

A social belief is a belief that is taught as being true. This type of belief comes from sources that are part of our social structure, such as parents, siblings, teachers, neighbours, strangers, media, advertising, books, classmates, peers, teachers, ministers, and/or anyone who may have instilled a belief in you that you believe to be true. In reality it may not be true. It may or may not be useful. It may not be authentic for you.

Notice your beliefs. Sometimes they fit with who you are. However, you may be driven by a belief, thinking that you need to do something because you should, instead of doing something because it feels true and right for you. Doing something because of a belief and a feeling of 'should do' can cause self-doubt, second guessing, inner dialogue, inner conflict, and perhaps anxiety. Noticing a belief helps us choose how to act. We may still follow a belief. However, at least we are aware that we are doing so.

Our brains lock onto beliefs because we have a deep-rooted need to belong. Going against a belief may mean risking exclusion. It is also noteworthy that we all have a combination of different beliefs. This can cause conflict within a family, a couple, or a community.

Cultural beliefs are passed down from generation to generation. When analyzed, they may have made sense four generations ago, but perhaps not now. Cultural beliefs come from our cultural heritage and families. Here are some examples:

✦   Canadians are known around the world as kind, gentle, and pleasant people. It is a generalization.

✦   Pre-marital sex: There are differences all over the world in how pre-marital sex is viewed. In some African tribal cultures, youths are encouraged to have multiple sexual partners before marriage to get the wandering urge out of their systems. Most North American parents do not condone sex amongst teens, although some help their teens practice safe sex, because they know that hormones are raging and teens will experiment. In many European countries sex is considered natural and part of human nature, so many families do not consider sexual relationships taboo. Many European women go topless on the beach. This is natural for them, and considered neither immodest nor a sexual provocation. A young woman visiting Canada bought a bathing suit top for the first time in her life. She found this strange.

✦ Death: Norms about death vary with each culture. The Chinese hire funeral criers to help people grieve. Mexicans celebrate the Day of the Dead, while North Americans tend to tidy up death with a closed casket, funeral and/or celebration of life, and move on. Embalming is a recent North American tradition that is not practiced throughout the world.

These are just a few examples of cultural differences.

I share this story in my workshops: A young girl asks her mother at Easter why the ham bone is removed and laid beside the ham. The mother answers, "I don't really know, my mother always did it that way. Let's ask her when she comes over for dinner." They ask the grandmother why the ham bone is cut out. She replied that that was how her mother always did it. She suggested it might be for flavour. Later that evening they visit Grannie and ask her if she knew why the ham bone was cut out. Grannie replied, "It was the only way the ham would fit in the wood stove."

Selected Common Beliefs

Life is dangerous.

You have to work hard for a living.

Opposites attract.

Boys are tough. Boys don't cry.

Girls are nice. It's ugly to be angry.

Canadians are gentle.

I make bad choices.

I'm ugly.

I am not relationship material.

Money is the root of all evil.

Rich people are crooks.

Blondes are dumb.

Blondes have more fun.

I'm not good enough.

Don't be too happy, in case something bad happens.

Skinny is beautiful.

Overweight people are lazy.

Good things don't come easy.

Play is frivolous.

Ask yourself if this belief is absolutely true 100% of the time. Then consider another perspective that may fit better for you and your situation.

6. Self-doubt

Self-doubt can be a symptom of low self esteem. The insecurity of second guessing, or back and forth questioning of a decision, and of being unaware of your authenticity, as well as conflict with beliefs, can create worry and anxiety.

Constant second guessing and self doubt can become a loop and create anxiety. The *Empowering Your Anxiety Warrior* section provides ideas to help you focus on learning to release self doubt and build your resilience, inner resources, and self esteem.

7. Perfectionism

Wanting to be right, to do everything correctly and to be perfect are other causes of much anxiety. To do our best, expect the best, and strive for the best are all integral goals. However, to be perfect as a parent, employee, artist, or student is unreasonable and a set-up for stress and anxiety. How can you be comfortable in the striving and imperfection? Can you be comfortable in the process? In the middle of a project? In the middle of completion? In the middle of the mess? Can a project or goal be partly finished and admired? Yes, to all of these questions.

Does perfectionism stop you from finishing a book? Building a house, writing a play, taking a course, learning how to paint?

8. Negative thinking

Take a moment to reflect on the quality of your thoughts. Do you mentally swear? Whether at traffic, or others, or yourself, or the weather? Is life fair? Does it feel like things are always going wrong?

Do you focus on mistakes? Flaws? Are you critical of others? Or perhaps, do you wonder why people are incompetent? Do you complain a lot? Do others say you complain a lot?

Negative thinking along with disaster thinking can perpetuate worry and anxiety.

We discuss the impact of language in points 10 and 11 of the chapter *Empowering Your Anxiety Warrior* (page 57-62). These sections show you how to be aware of language and how to change language so that it reflects your dreams and desires.

Can you consider inconveniences as opportunities? Challenges as learning curves?

9. High sensitivity

A highly sensitive person (*HSP*), also known as a person with sensory processing sensitivity (SPS), is someone who is hypersensitive to external stimuli and who has a greater depth of cognitive processing and high emotional reactivity. These terms were popularized in the mid-1990s by Elaine Aron. SPS is measured by the Highly Sensitive Person Scale (HSPS), developed by Aron.

According to Aron and colleagues (1997), people with high SPS comprise about 15% to 20% of the population. These people are thought to process sensory data more deeply due to the nature of their central nervous systems. Aron and colleagues state that high SPS is not a disorder and that it is associated with both positive and negative attributes.

Having high sensitivity as a character trait can make one more susceptible to anxiety and/or feeling overwhelmed. Those of us who are highly sensitive need to take care of our sensitivity. It is imperative that we have as resources daily practice and grounding skills.

The Highly Sensitive Child

In my private practice I see many highly sensitive children. Is your child highly attuned to his or her senses? Does he or she have an excellent sense of smell or hearing? React more to pain?

Is your child easily overwhelmed emotionally? Or likely to withdraw when over-stimulated?

Many of my young clients want to hide in bed under the covers.

Perhaps your son has a greater depth of understanding than his peers, or even adults. Does he ask profound questions, think a lot on his own, or reflect on his experiences?

Is your daughter highly aware of her surroundings? Does she notice when small household items are moved, or minor changes in others, like a haircut?

Is your child very sensitive to other people's emotions? Does he or she notice when someone is feeling sad and try to help? Or appear to be especially sensitive to the feelings of animals?

If this sounds like your child, learn more about raising a sensitive child at: www.education.com/magazine/article/Raising_Sensitive_Child/

10. Memories

We've all experienced smells, actions, colours, touches, tastes, and sounds that trigger wonderful memories. That's because our long-term memory is linked to parts of the brain that regulate our emotional and physical reactions to situations and events. But if these sensory triggers are connected to stressful situations or events, they may cause anxiety. Sometimes just the trigger alone can cause anxiety, without us even recalling the memory.

11. Traumas

If you have experienced a recent trauma, processing it will take time. During this period it is natural to feel some anxiety. This anxiety will lessen over a few weeks until it disappears, but sometimes the brain gets backed up. Big and small traumas can get stuck when the brain has not processed, or cannot process, the trauma. This can happen over time or it can happen with one incident or multiple traumas.

A small trauma, a 'small t', could result from falling over a bike, having to get stitches, or being falsely accused of stealing. A big trauma, a 'big T', is catastrophic, like a car accident, a fire, combat, a death, and so on. The brain is equipped to process trauma, but sometimes it can't. Sometimes the reasons are clear, other times not. When the brain cannot process the trauma, this is called post-traumatic stress. As mentioned previously in the discussion of possible post-traumatic stress, seeking professional help may be advisable.

Check-in

Here is another good time to use the check-in scale. What is your level of anxiety, from 0 to 10? Are some of the layers previously mentioned manageable? Are you curious? Then continue reading, as the rest of the book is about resources and strategies to empower your warrior.

Empowering Your Anxiety Warrior

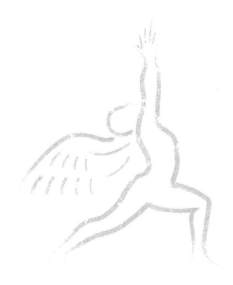

Empowering Your Anxiety Warrior

This section of this book is full of strategies to fight anxiety, based on my own exploration of anxiety and my work with clients. Try, explore, and play. Discover the strategies you like and those that give you the most energy. There will be times when you may need only one, or several. Everyone is different, and every episode of anxiety could be different. Pick and choose the strategies that work for you. Some activities will weave together with other activities. Others stand alone.

In my talks and in this book, I emphasize the importance of being aware, noticing, and practicing.

Life is practice, mastery is practice, gratitude is practice. Managing anxiety is practice, too.

Consider how you are going to create your own daily practice techniques.

In my personal journal I have compiled a list of strategies that I know from experience work for me: grounding, breathing, gratitude practice, bubble shield, step back/watch, pause, notice, safe place meditation, container, affirmations, setting mindful intentions, creating positive beliefs that work for me, singing bowl vibrations, positive movies, journaling, nature, walks, snowshoeing, kayaking, gardening, cycling, comedies, laughter, playing, being well rested (sleeping well, taking naps), good nutrition, social connections (I am an introvert and sometimes need to stretch myself to be social), yoga, massage, tapping, energy group, silent mediation. Many of these strategies appear below.

When I need to, I refer to my list. I invite you to create a list for yourself based on the strategies presented here. Mix and match and adjust to suit your needs. Have your list handy in several places. When we are anxious it may be near impossible to think about what we need, but simple to remember where our list is.

Whatever your 'combination' is, make it your own and practice it daily. My clients and I notice an improvement in the quality of life: we feel less anxious, more positive and happier.

**The more connected you are to yourself,
the more connected you are to your world.**

Strategies

1. Mastering your mind

You always have a choice. You can choose to think happy, positive, constructive thoughts and go to those memory banks where you were joyful and strong. You can choose to focus on the gifts and the opportunities of life. Or you can choose a path of negativity and focus on what you do not have.

Be aware of your thought patterns, and how the same thoughts can repeat many times. Push them away by self-prompts, such as saying, "Next!".

Journal writing is very helpful in processing new thoughts. For more about this, see the journaling exercises on pages 71-75. Decide what you want to experience and take steps to support that decision.

You are not your brain

When something triggered my anxiety, I thought it was me. I thought my brain was the same thing as my mind. I didn't realize that they are different. Then I took a step back and began to explore how the brain reacts, what causes pathological anxiety, and how we can overcome it to become happier.

For me, these reactions had presented a mystery. We know that we can think differently, but we generally don't. We know that we can 'change channels', yet we generally don't.

Deepak Chopra and the National Science Foundation say that we have about 50,000 to 70,000 thoughts a day, most of which are repetitive. Part of their function is to keep our minds active and sane, and partly they are our belief systems at work.

What is the brain's function? This main internal computer runs the whole body. The brain makes us breathe, beats our heart, has fevers, collects data, learns, has looping thoughts, reactions, triggers, and habits, all to keep us alive.

Many things affect the brain before 'we' (our minds) get involved. What if I showed you that you are not your brain? What if I showed you a way to be the master of your brain?

Your brain needs your help. Your brain needs you to be the master, and needs you to partner with it and its functions.

Your brain is the first organ to form in utero. From the moment it forms, it begins collecting information: data, history, memories, patterns, and senses. It collects social and cultural beliefs, generational beliefs both positive and negative, and information on how to direct and signal the body and keep it functioning.

As it collects information via the eyes, ears, and other sensory organs, the brain learns and memorizes. It controls motor functions and balances the body's digestion, healing, fevers, mending, and breathing. With this data, the brain learns and forms responses and reactions.

You and I mostly are not aware of this collecting. Imagine babies and toddlers. These young humans do not filter or articulate various beliefs, nor are they able to discern the information their brains receive.

How to expand the joy space in your brain

Sometimes our brains have more unpleasant memories than happy ones, whether due to circumstances or habit. I call this the 'pain space'. When our pain space is bigger than our joy space it becomes the default thinking pattern. Even when the brain has a happy experience, the default neuropathways lead the way to the pain space and we experience the same symptoms as pain or trauma — nervous stomach, trembling, insomnia, a sense of flatness, numbness, loss of appetite, and so on.

Here are ways in which we can expand our joy space:

+ Blessing people.

+ Praying.

+ Forgiving.

✦ Practicing gratitude.

✦ Sharing grace.

✦ Loving — the process of life, beauty, being alive,
  another person, knowledge, pets.

✦ Accepting the miracles of our bodies, other animals,
  plants, trees, the universe, the planet Earth, stars.

✦ Remembering fun things.

✦ Recalling good memories.

✦ Repeating good things.

✦ Enjoying comedy and jokes; laughter.

Why this works

The brain can learn new habits and change itself. The brain relates to
the familiar; for instance, when you get a new car, you notice the same
models on the roads. If you buy a certain make of running shoes, you
tend to notice other people wearing a similar shoe. If you're a parent-
to-be you find yourself smiling and nodding at expectant mothers.

You can change your inner dialogue to a new familiar of; oppor-
tunity-thinking, manifesting your dreams, experiencing miracles and
seeing the wonder of life and this universe.

Become the master of your brain, pause, step back, and take
charge. Partner with your brain. It got you this far with what it has
gathered. With awareness you can give it other options and strategies
to cope with anxiety.

Awareness:
How can you change what
you are not aware of?

Check out your mental blocks

If you are not aware of your thoughts, how can you change them?
Become aware of your perceptions, assumptions, suppositions, beliefs,
prejudices, and judgments/point of view. I am not saying you need to

decide whether a perception is right or wrong, it is simply your perception. Be aware of it and notice that you use this as a lens to see your life through. Be clear that it is your perception, not another's. Someone else has other perceptions/point of views. Once you can identify a perception, ask yourself: Does it cause you or others discomfort or pain? Does this point of view hold you back from thriving? If it does, it might be wise to either accept your perception as your own and/or to modify your perception.

Earlier we looked at some social and cultural beliefs, so let's look now at some various blocks to moving forward and progressing.

Do any of the blocks below seem familiar? If you have noticed some of your own. I invite you to open up your thinking and creativity and consider alternatives, to allow flow and moving forward.

Belief systems that can block your progress

"Play is frivolous."

"To err is wrong."

"I'm not creative."

"I'm not smart."

"Follow the rules."

"Don't be foolish — this is not practical."

"It costs too much."

"I don't have time for that."

Some of these can be very strong. Some are deeply embedded from childhood, our culture, and our family. These beliefs may be very resistant to moving aside or going away. One way to manage them is to notice them, greet them, embrace them, understand them, maybe work with them. What challenges do they present? What opportunities and strengths could they bring?

Blocks to creativity

Negative beliefs that create a lack of confidence, a sense of competitiveness, unrealistic expectations, and blocked emotions can all inhibit creativity. Conflicting beliefs can cause self-doubt and second guessing. As we move along in this book, a few different approaches will be presented.

Negative beliefs

When you were growing up, did you ever hear, "Your sister has all the artistic talent in the family," or, "You don't have the body of a dancer," or "You sing off key"? These and many other negative comments can shut you down in your creative pursuits.

Often, as parents, we can be career-focused for our children and think that if they do not have enough talent for a career, then it is pointless for them to pursue their love of just being creative. We forget how important this pursuit may be to their future livelihoods. Growing up, a child remembers those negative comments, but not always where they came from. As adults, we believe we are not capable of drawing or dancing, writing, or sculpting, and should not 'waste our time' if we will not be good at it. Sometimes, after many years, my clients come to me, scared yet driven, to reawaken and nurture what was pushed away in their youth. Many others don't even try, believing that they have no aptitude at all, and that there is no sense in making the effort.

What cynical onlooker has not asked, "What are you wasting your time on? Isn't there something worthwhile you can do?" Such thoughtless comments can be crushing.

In *Creative Practices*, number 1 (page 131), explore your own list of mental blocks.

2. Starting a mental checklist of anxiety triggers

In my personal life, as well as in my professional practice, I have learned that I need to check in with myself — my body, mind, spirit, and emotions. When I have anxiety, I start working through a mental checklist of possible anxiety triggers.

For instance, I've learned that if I wake up with anxiety, it could be a sign of dehydration. If this is the case, within minutes of drinking water the anxious feeling goes away.

If the anxiety persists, I begin looking at what is on my schedule. Too many things to do? Stress-related events? Deadlines? Something exciting?

To reduce the anxiety, I do some grounding exercises, such as slower breathing, or the Brain Gym Hook-Up described in the chapter on *Brain Fitness: For a Fit Brain and a Fit Life* (page 109), or perhaps take a walk or do some yoga. I also begin some self-talk and journaling. These are just some of the items on my personal list of strategies. Sometimes I need to resort to essential oils such as lavender and to the Bach Flower Rescue Remedy (page 68).

My mental checklist

I've reproduced my mental checklist below. Start one for yourself. First, ask yourself, what are my symptoms? Headaches, tense shoulders, localized pain, nausea, shaking, heart pain?

Is the cause physical?

+ Have I slept enough?

+ Do I need water?

+ Is the cause a substance? What did I ingest? What did I eat yesterday?

+ Is the cause external?

+ Am I wearing my proper glasses? (Sometimes I wear magnifiers.)

+ Am I excited? Sometimes I am so excited my body feels anxious.

+ What is on my agenda? Have I piled far too many things on myself? Has life?

+ What are my thoughts; kind and loving, or critical?

+ Am I over stimulated?

When asking myself these questions, I'm really working through the eleven layers of anxiety described earlier (pages 17 to 27). It's a helpful starting point for creating your own mental checklist.

3. Listening to your body's sensations

Listening to your body can take many forms. It may involve sensations, images, or visions, as well as emotions.

Body focusing is a way of listening to your body. Appreciate that your body remembers everything, is programmed for survival, and is constantly attempting to communicate to you what it requires.

We trust our body and brain to maintain our temperature. If it is slightly out of line, we do not feel well and sense something is not right. As babies and children, we were very much in tune with our bodies. We made our demands known without inhibition, as every parent knows. As we grew older, judgment, pressure, criticism, intimidation, and negation may have taught us to discredit those feelings or to judge them as wrong or unimportant, and thus question them, disregard or submerge them.

When you feel uncharacteristically tired or out of sorts, pay attention to the feeling and slow down. Again, listen to what your inner voice has to say.

Ignoring these body sensations or pushing them away does not make them go away. These sensations get stuffed somewhere in the body and reappear by surprise when triggered in some way, usually when we least expect a reaction. This is a set-up for disease and discomfort.

It's healthier to accept and confront bodily sensations. We need to acknowledge them, experience them, and deal with them if we can.

When something is worrying you, when you feel hurt or angry, take some quiet time to sort out what is really bothering you. Talk to yourself or write in a journal. When that is not enough, talk with a good friend or someone close. Expressing yourself through painting, poetry, and/or music helps bring the feeling outside of yourself. Release the discomfort.

Try to sense the source of your feelings. For example, your sickly stomach could be a warning, indicating nervousness, anxiety, or fear. A cold could indicate that you are run down and need rest. Headaches could indicate eye strain, tension, stress, worry, or uneasiness, or dehydration. Certain pains are alert signals. Get to know and trust your body. Note if any trouble seems to last. If you can't put a finger on the source, check it out with your health practitioner.

When something is unbalanced, your body knows it and immediately sets out to balance, repair, and heal itself. Your body is constantly checking in and adjusting itself to maintain this equilibrium.

As you practice noticing the more obvious and stronger shifts in energy, you will be able to tune into the more subtle energy shifts within you.

Sometimes habits don't feel good anymore, and we may need to let them go, or perhaps even certain people or their behaviours.

As we practice noticing our energy levels, we can recognize our body's cues and naturally gravitate to things that we enjoy more. We also learn to conserve our energy, protect it and nurture it. We can learn to thrive again. I have learned that when I work with passion and joy, I have so much energy.

Learn more on how to read and strengthen your body's clues with the 'Yes/no/maybe' exercise in the *Creative Practices*, number 6 (page 137).

4. Listening to your inner voice

Is it your body talking? Or your inner voice? It may be different for each of you and it may be different in various situations. As you do the exercises, build your daily practice and gain awareness, your inner check-in and awareness will become clearer.

Your feelings are accurate indicators of balance and rightness in your life. When you have a feeling — uneasy or pleasant — about a place, a person, or even an idea, pay attention to the feeling and check it out. Ask yourself why this feeling is happening. Listen objectively to your inner voice.

> **By becoming sensitive to your inner voice, you will begin hearing the many layers of possibilities, memories, experiences, habits, and love and fears that can influence that inner voice.**

Suppressing or denying feelings and body sensations — whether pleasant or unpleasant — can cause them to become hostages to your body and your mind. As time passes, these suppressed feelings may find expression in confused emotions. Over time, muddled feelings and misunderstood emotions can severely impact our ability to have healthy relationships and live a healthy, balanced life.

By consciously striving to develop an awareness of how you truly feel about something, actively acknowledging how you feel will lower the intensity of those feelings. Taking time to sit with these feelings will clarify or dissipate them.

Expressing your feelings freely by participating in the arts, music, drama, movement, visual arts, and creative writing can help to discharge feelings safely and non-verbally, making way for clearer thinking and calmer emotions.

To strengthen your inner voice and inner understanding, begin to notice when you feel lighter or heavier, constricted or elated. As you recall a favourite pet making you laugh, perhaps a good friend calling on you, or your grandchildren, notice your energy shift. Think of a time you were on your 'A' game. Notice how your body feels.

Then shift to a not-so-good time in your life, perhaps when you felt embarrassed, or felt like you were failing. Perhaps you were caught off guard at something. Notice your body. How is this feeling different from when you laugh or smile?

Notice how a dog plays: they have no reason or direction, they do it for sheer joy. Ever watch a bird soar, dip and dive, and catch the wind? Sometimes it's just for the pleasure of the act.

Have you ever noticed a room that feels particularly comfortable? Or, in contrast, entered a room where, perhaps the air is so thick with tension you could cut it with a knife, as the saying goes? We have all felt this at one time or another. This is your inner knowing, sometimes called intuition or gut feeling. At times you may experience many feelings at once.

Ask yourself, "Where are these feelings coming from?", "What options are open to me?", "Is this the best answer for me?", "Is it the best answer for my life? My family? My community?" When contemplating our lives and choices, such reflective questions can help us to change old patterns and dramas that replay in our lives.

Ask yourself if that inner answer is based on fear or denial, or is truly in your best interest. Sometimes there is more than one level to an answer. Listen to them all and put them in their place.

✦ What would your answer be, coming from a feeling of love?

✦ What would your answer be, coming from a feeling of fear?

✦ Try journaling or discussing that 'inner voice' with a supportive friend.

✦ To really listen, be still.

By consciously striving to develop an awareness of how you really feel about something, and taking time to think about it, you will clarify or dissipate confused or conflicting feelings. The section on 'Making decisions' (page 49) may also assist in this thinking process.

5. Caring for your physical self

I have included this section on physical self-care as it is one of the first places where we can identify what needs to be changed. This section does not replace diet books or books dedicated to self-care, such as *Brain Fitness: For a Fit Brain and a Fit Life*, which includes many practical suggestions. Many times, I have found that when I change my environments or self care, my anxiety and stress levels decrease. Stress is subjective. It can evoke excitement and challenge, and it can also invoke illness, exhaustion, and despair. I intend to give my body the best fuel I can and the best care, so it can be as resilient as possible for life.

Assess your working and home environment. Is your body being stressed from second-hand smoke, pollution, noise, fumes, water chemical treatments, inadequate or harsh lighting, variations in air pressure, stale air, or other chemicals such as perfumes, cleaners and solvents?

We cannot control all elements in our world, but some stresses can be eliminated or managed. Do what you can. Remember that each negative experience weakens you, just as every positive one strengthens you.

Look after your physical body

This is where you live. If this body breaks down, where else are you going to live?

It makes sense that a healthy body will have more energy and vitality. A healthy body is important for a healthy mind, just as a healthy mind is important for a healthy body. Machinery mistreated or lacking repairs breaks down in time. Like any machine, your body needs proper maintenance, fuel, and care. The following points are a simple invitation for you to consider the well-being of your physical body. If any of these resonate with you, it is an invitation to pursue this further.

Eat right

Healthy food is imperative for happy, balanced, creative living. Quality food must be a priority. To function well, our bodies need fresh foods free of pesticides, hormones, and additives. Continued weariness and lack of energy could be caused by poor diet and artificial stimulants. How much processed sugar and caffeine are in your diet? In *Brain Fitness: For a Fit Brain and a Fit Life* (page 101), Jill Hewlett says more.

Eating on the run, in your car, choosing fast food and eating in a hurry, can add stress and create anxiety in the body. Eating too much and not chewing food properly stresses your digestive system. Drinking too much fluid puts a strain on your stomach by diluting stomach acid and digestive enzymes.

Drink water

That said, it is nonetheless important to drink a minimum of 14 ounces (about two cups or half a litre) of water per day. Your body, especially the kidneys and liver, needs water to help flush toxins from your system. Tea and other liquids are not the same as plain, clear, delicious water. Your body doesn't need to filter water and can flush toxins more easily and quickly with water than with other liquids. Your body needs water, and as mentioned before, will give you anxiety-like symptoms when dehydrated.

> *Case study:* Recently, a client came in suffering from anxiety and long-term depression. After we chatted for a while, I began sharing some simple information about physical and chemical substances that affect the brain. One of the things we noted was that she did not drink enough water. In her next visit, she reported that she now drinks a glass of water at waking and carries a water bottle with her in order to drink more during the day. She reported that she was amazed on how much better she felt, even though her life circumstances had not changed much in a week.

Exercise

Exercise for energy. This doesn't mean becoming an athlete. It means keeping active with walks, bicycle riding, swimming, tai chi, yoga, dancing, playing with children or grandchildren, gardening, stretching, or working. Keeping all your parts agile and moving easily keeps you in shape for most of the activities and expectations of your life. Exercise stimulates happiness and well-being. If you are feeling low, take a brisk one-hour walk and notice the difference in how you feel.

Rest

Are you getting enough sleep? Good sleep means restful, uninterrupted sleep. If you could sleep as long as you liked, how long would you sleep? Do you regularly drag yourself out of bed when summoned by your alarm clock, and stimulate your body with caffeine to get going? How often do you consume sugar-loaded or refined foods during the day for energy? Listen to your body.

Are you suffering from insomnia? Is stress making you sleepless? Or is the insomnia stressing your body? Insomnia has different causes, such as diet, medical or social problems, trauma, environment, stimulants, over-tiredness, and alcohol consumption. Listen to your body for clues. Investigate your reactions to the possible causes. For me, I find that chocolate, any amount of caffeine, the computer, terrifying movies before bed, and exciting plans ahead are triggers for my restless nights.

Try some relaxation techniques. Regular exercise also helps promote sound sleep. See what works for you. To increase your energy, look at your passions: when you are passionate about what you do or have in your life, you will have energy.

Brush your skin

Skin is the body's largest organ, so skin care is important for optimum health. Dry brushing your skin daily removes dead skin flakes. By dry brushing your skin you help it to breathe, and toxins are released more readily.

Use a natural bristle body brush or a dry stiff loofah sponge. Gently brush in circular motions, moving up the body. You will feel tingly, alive, and refreshed. Let your skin breathe further by putting only natural, breathable fabrics next to it.

**Caring for our physical body
enhances our mental state
and our general health.**

You are a priority

It is hard to be balanced when you are fuelled on junk food and stimulants, and lack sleep. Physical depletion affects the mental and emotional capabilities of the mind.

Make caring for yourself a priority. Your body is the only one you have and it has to last a lifetime. Nurture yourself by building and supporting the person you are. Believe in yourself, look after your needs, and you will thrive. As you nourish, heal, encourage, and comfort yourself, you will be more able to give the same to others. It is our responsibility to look after our needs.

Your emerging happiness and actions will touch everything in your daily life. The energy you exude can ripple through to your family, your neighbourhood, and your community. Sliding along on the surface, staying in your habits and not challenging yourself or looking after yourself, may seem like an easier road, but it can get a little slimy too.

To embrace life is fulfilling and terrifying all at once, but always worth it.

Humour and play

Have a laugh during the day. Read some comic books, make a laugh list, watch a funny movie, collect favourite cartoons and decorate your workplace. Have fun!

Too often, we become bunged up in our routine or task, taking ourselves too seriously. Then we forget where we came from and what we really are doing here. Humour frees us up. It heals and lightens our load.

Play is magnanimous. Play is healing. Laughter is healing.

**Play and fun are powerful motivators
for creative thought and genius. Play
loosens, livens and opens us up.**

Play gives us a break from serious routine.

Take time to play. You, your family, and your work will benefit. Ideas will pop out of your brain while you are frolicking in the water, chasing your children around the house, or playing tag with your dog. Maybe it's a hobby; beading, cooking, gardening? What brings you joy? Laughter?

Try it. You'll like it and you'll be productive. Really!

Make your own laugh list

Here's what makes me laugh:

- ✦ My dog proudly carrying a stick eight times his length.

- ✦ Tickling my son.

- ✦ Dancing *in the rain*.

- ✦ Making up a language and asking people for directions.

- ✦ Eating without utensils.

- ✦ Popping popcorn without a lid on the pot.

- ✦ Watching a baby eat chocolate pudding.

Creative holiday

For those stress triggers over which you and I have little control, a dose of creativity helps to lighten the mood, change the scene, and refresh the mind. Shifting to a creative activity for a time is like shifting gears. It can also help return you to your 'normal' self. A period of creativity can be as rejuvenating as a nap.

> **Experiencing the arts — music, dance, painting, and so on — can help the body and mind transcend blocked emotions and memories, and lessen tension and stressful periods.**

Do you feel stuck?

Freeing yourself up creatively can add passion to your life, release energy, and lessen anxiety. Do you feel creatively stifled, trapped? Becoming aware of your mental traps is the first step to getting free of them.

+ Ask yourself: How practical am I? Is being practical a priority?

+ Do you see your work routine as logical, cost-effective, and/or boring?

+ What if I tried something out of the ordinary today? Would it feel crazy? Out of control? What would happen?

Try not to be judgmental of your new ideas or different actions. Mix one day up, as a holiday from your routine. Have some fun. You will have changed your energy flow.

Do you always follow the rules of procedure, the guidelines for techniques, or the same order in your work? Break a pattern, break any one pattern or break a lot of them.

Challenge yourself.

+ Do a task in a different order.

+ What would your problem (or task) look like from someone else's perspective? How would you look if you were performing your task while holding a banana? Play it through in your mind. Sometimes a silly or funny idea can break us out of our seriousness.

+ Try something new.

+ Learn a new skill, then practice it.

+ Risk feeling foolish, or just looking foolish. Risk having fun.

+ Dream up a new possibility. Ask yourself, "What if?"

There is not just one approach. Avoid investing in only one inspiration. Know that there are many 'right' approaches. People who know me hear me say, "There are many roads to Rome."

One of my favourite teachers, Bill Bayley, asked us for 10 solutions to a design problem. When the whole class moaned, he reminded us that there are hundreds of approaches to that particular design problem alone. He saw that each time he handed out the same exercise, year after year.

Solutions, innovations, transformations, and ideas are all out there. Let's discover and develop them. Be open to them.

Life is a smorgasbord

Some days you may just want dessert. Some days you want meat and potatoes. Some days you want to try everything.

Appetite fluctuates. Honour your appetite. In everything that you do — workshops, practices, techniques, beliefs — choose from the smorgasbord of life and assemble your plate to suit your tastes and appetite for today.

Don't hesitate to explore, learn, study, and grow in unexpected ways, and at different times. Sometimes you need to explore with your intuition and sometimes you may want a guide. Listen to yourself and to what you need. Ask yourself, why does everything in life need to stay the same?

Nature

Nature is all around us, even in the cities, in the trees, and birds and weather. Nature is intrinsic to who we are, and to our relationships to plants, animals, and other features of the planet. Humans have a need to connect with nature. When we are in nature, our own biological rhythms attune to nature's rhythms.

Connecting and being in nature is grounding and healthy. Many studies show that the closer you are to nature and green spaces, the happier you feel. Nature actually changes your brain. When you take a walk, electrochemical changes occur in your brain, producing calming and favourable results. I find personally that I might begin a walk, anxious or stressed, and by the end of my walk I am thinking more clearly and calmly. The sights and sounds of nature are relaxing to the mind and body.

When it is sunny, no matter how cold the weather or where I am, I try to face the sun and catch some rays of Vitamin D. Again, studies have shown that even a few minutes of sunshine will keep our mood elevated. Vitamin D helps prevent disease and infection, and is essential to bone health. It is also a feel-good vitamin that helps prevent Seasonal Affective Disorder (SAD). This is also known as winter depression, winter blues, or seasonal depression.

Case study: A few winters ago, the season was particularly long and cloudy. My friends and colleagues and I, who are usually positive and upbeat, were wearing down. I was lamenting to a dear colleague about how low I felt. She suggested using a sunlamp, which provides the same spectrum of light as the sun. I ordered one and installed it on top of my desk, which does not get much natural light. Within three days, I was surprised to find that I felt better.

Fresh air and exposure to nature also help you sleep. Sunshine in the morning helps set your internal biological clock to sleep at night.

Being outside in nature is good for your mental health. Being in nature usually means some kind of physical exercise. Try it for yourself and listen to your body.

6. Making decisions

Decision making can create a lot of anxiety, especially if you second-guess yourself and want to make the 'right' decision. I used to think that I would know the 'right' decision because it would feel good. I learned it is not always so. Sometimes the choice is between feeling badly or less badly. A good friend once said that sometimes we need to choose the way that causes the least discomfort. Not every decision has a happy ending.

It is not unusual to have mixed feelings regarding any personal decision. These mixed feelings can create confusion, hesitation, or an overwhelmed sensation. Even once a decision has been made, second guessing and self doubt can creep in. Some decisions have many layers.

Most decisions can be done in steps. Usually, our initial impulse is the 'right' one. Still yourself and try and remember your first impulse.

Take your time to understand the layers so you can make a choice with the most clarity possible.

When I read the following excerpt on decision making in Dr. Susan Jeffers' book, *Feel the Fear and Do It Anyway*, it immediately caught my attention. She suggests that we cannot make any poor decisions. When I read this, I thought Dr. Jeffers had written this chapter for me. I was so impressed with this model, I share it often with my clients. The following paraphrases Dr. Jeffers' advice, with my insights added.

No-lose decision-making process

Before making a decision,

1. Use affirmations like "I will do fine no matter what decision I make. Golden opportunities are everywhere. I will look forward to the opportunities of learning and growing that either choice gives me." Practice positive thinking exercises and affirmations.

2. Research your decision, product, purchase, trip etc... It's okay to gather feedback, however, consider it with all your research.

3. Establish your priorities. (I learned that each decision has a different set of priorities.)

4. Trust your body sense and intuition. Trust your gut. Your body will give you clues and a sense of what feels better.

5. Lighten up and do not take each decision so seriously. Usually, a decision is really not that important. Glean whatever you can from life lessons.

After making a decision,

1. Throw away your expectations. We cannot control every outcome, no matter how much we prepare and organize. You might be disappointed if you expect a certain outcome, and you may miss any unexpected benefits and opportunities.

2. Accept total responsibility for making the decision. Sometimes in our society we look to blame another person if the decision does not work out the way we want. Know that no one forced your hand.

3. Don't protect, correct. I remember having much angst over a particular decision. When I made it, I was committed to sticking to it no matter how painful it became. It never occurred to me that I could reverse my decision and change direction. Even after good research and sincere thoughtfulness, a decision may not turn out to be what you hoped. It is okay to notice and then change your mind and take a new direction. How else are we going to know if the decision is the one we want? Sometimes a decision may need modifying. We need to try it out. And we can learn. A decision is not a failure; it is a try.

Now, I am more at ease with decisions. If a decision feels disappointing, inadequate or unsettling somehow, it may mean that I need to take the time to regroup and to modify the decision as needed. I am more relaxed and not as anxious.

The above makes total sense, though this is not what we usually do, me included!

No-win decision-making process

Before making a decision,

1. Focus on a No-Win Model; worry about all the things that could go wrong. Let negative thinking overtake your thoughts, making sure it will be a disaster, making certain that you will make the wrong decision, that all of your effort is a waste of time.

2. Try to predict and control the future. Paralyze yourself with anxiety.

3. Go against your authentic self, don't trust your intuition and listen to what everyone else thinks.

4. Let the burden of decision making ruin your day.

After making a decision,

1. Try to micro-manage the outcome, try to control all the elements around you.

2. If the decision does not bring you what you want, wallow in angst about it, blame others for distracting you, blame others for influencing you, blame nature; anything to justify that you are upset and disappointed.

3. If your decision is successful, wonder if it would have been better the other way.

Do you protect a decision that went poorly? After all, there is so much invested, so perhaps you should suffer instead.

Did you know that airplanes on autopilot fly off course 90% of the time? They are constantly auto-correcting on autopilot. Dr. Jeffers introduces this model as an example of how to negotiate our decisions, knowing our goals and auto correcting/fine tuning as we need to, as life changes all around us.

OFF-COURSE/CORRECT MODEL

7. Using affirmations

The word 'affirmation' comes from the Latin *affirmare*, originally meaning 'to make steady, strengthen'. Daily affirmations are positive phrases that you create to describe how you want to be in your life.

I use the Internet to access free daily inspirational quotes. There are many to choose from, with various themes. These inspirations begin a train of thought that guides my thinking in an inspired way. I also have many favourite authors who wrote great inspirational books. I regularly use these quotes to create new affirmations. They are very effective when practiced daily. Doing so conditions our brains to adopt similar positive messages and ways of thinking. Our brains relate to what is familiar in our world. Even though an affirmation may feel false in the beginning, as your brain slowly relaxes into the familiarity of the positive message it begins to feel that it is possible and real.

Be very careful with your words, choosing to speak only those that work towards your well-being.

Thoughts have power and energy. When we change our thoughts, we restructure the neural pathways of our brains. When we think we are victims, that is what we will be. When we think we are creative, then we are creative.

Affirmations do indeed strengthen our brains by helping them believe in the potential of an action we want to come true. When we write these same affirmations, they become even stronger. Much like exercise, the more you exercise your brain, the stronger it becomes. The level of feel-good hormones rises and pushes our brains to form new clusters of positive thoughts and stronger neuropathways.

If you constantly say, "I can't," the energy of your words will indeed set you up to not be able. When you say, "I can!", the energy of your words will do just that. Our thoughts translate into words. Eventually those words translate into actions.

Be a wordsmith: be aware of your language and choose carefully the words that will help you to make your intentions manifest.

The words will become familiar and eventually a self-fulfilling prophecy and your reality. Using positive affirmations gives you back control of your mind and the information it receives. It puts you in the driver's seat and lets you flood it with positive information that will change you for the better.

Here are examples of positive affirmations for confidence. Modify them to suit yourself by using your own words:

+ I am a naturally confident person.

+ I can joyously be myself.

+ I am confident socially and enjoy meeting new people.

+ I am confident at all times and in all areas of my life.

+ Confidence comes naturally to me.

+ Being naturally self-confident and comfortable within myself is part of who I am.

8. Staying present: Breathing

A useful skill for managing anxiety to be present in the moment, self-aware, and noticing your environment. To do this we need to slow down, and/or pause. Mindful breathing helps us to do this and to be more present.

Everyone breathes. In fact, you probably only become aware of your breathing when attention is called to it. But did you know that learning to breathe well is important for your physical, emotional, and mental health?

Deep breathing is a powerful relaxant as well as a rejuvenator.

Breathing slowly lowers heart rate, metabolic rate, and blood pressure, and eases muscle tension. Breathing deeply and slowly cleanses, refreshes, detoxifies by removing carbon dioxide, and energizes mind and body.

Becoming aware of your breathing and taking time for deep-breathing exercises brings you in tune with your body, and also provides energy and calmness for deliberate and productive thinking. By slowing down and calming down, our intuition becomes clearer and stronger.

Children breathe naturally and deeply. Somehow, we adults have unlearned this.

+ Today, notice how many times you hold your breath.

+ Each time you think of it, breathe deeply at least three times.

+ Sit, stand, or, if possible, lie down. Keep your spine straight so you can feel your belly move.

+ Do not cross any limbs. Feel loose. Relax.

+ Gently place your fingers slightly interlaced and barely touching on your abdomen, resting on your navel. As you inhale through your nose into the depths of your lungs, allow your stomach to expand and push your fingers apart.

✦ Exhale slowly through your mouth, pushing out as
   much air as possible.

✦ Repeat several times.

Once this feels comfortable, try exhaling from the bottom of your
spine, pushing all the air out of your system. Open your mouth in a
relaxed fashion and notice how air naturally comes into your lungs.
Exhale again. Be patient; the sensation is subtle. The breathing
becomes the action of exhaling only and the air comes in naturally
on its own to fill the empty lungs.

**Whatever you are doing, try to be aware of how
you are breathing. Enjoy your breathing.**

Allow yourself time to focus only on your breathing, as outlined in
Creative Practices, number 8, 'Getting in Touch with Your Breathing'
(page 138).

Sometimes, unfamiliar experiences feel uncomfortable at first, like
writing with your non-dominate hand or sleeping on the other side
of the bed. Discomfort sometimes shows up as tiredness, giggles or
boredom. After you have tried these new things a few times, they
become comfortable and familiar. Like any skill, breathing properly
takes practice. In the meantime, you benefit right away, building
your overall health.

**Whenever you think about breathing,
straighten your back, drop your shoulders,
and consciously breathe deeply a few times.**

For three different breathing exercises that take only minutes to
perform, see *Creative Practices*, numbers 8 to 12 (pages 138 to 141).

There are also many forms of moving and breathing exercises and
relaxation exercises; for example, yoga, tai chi, qigong, and mindful
walking. Enjoy a new awareness of your breathing and your body.

9. Staying present: Meditating

Meditation can take many forms and serve many purposes. It can
be performed as a momentary stress reliever or as a way of life. In
meditation,

✦ You bring your awareness to your mind and your thoughts, you become aware of your thinking, and rest here.

✦ You let go of worry, fears, distress, and pain. Clear your mind of any desire. As you let go of these tensions, your heart will sense confidence and your understanding will grow.

Meditation can be described as:

Being present

Being aware.

Being awake.

Paying attention to life.

Understanding and watching.

Stopping awhile to listen.

Meditation can help you be more thoughtful and more in control of your thoughts. Meditation can help relieve stress, and is used for pain management. By getting to know yourself in meditation you can be in charge of your happiness.

Often my clients worry about meditating 'correctly'. They think their minds must be empty of thought. Because we have minds, we're always going to have thoughts and emotions. Much of the time our minds run unleashed and wild. We can be easily distracted by what's around us, or by chatter in our heads.

Sometimes, when I begin to meditate, it feels impossible to slow my mind down. However, the very action of trying to slow down or unwind is beneficial. Meditation does not eliminate thought, but instead helps us reflect and consider the thought by eliminating chatter. As our minds relax and our thoughts slow down, the spaces between thoughts become longer. Lengthening these gaps is the real work of meditation.

Meditation can take many forms. The chapter on *Creative Practices*, numbers 11 and 12 (pages 141 to 143) discusses two forms, moving and sitting.

How long do I need to sit meditatively?

Entering a state of mindfulness is less about the length of time than the quality of time. Five minutes of wakeful practice is more valuable than 20 minutes of dozing.

Begin practicing with short sessions. Restless, busy thoughts will inevitably intrude. When this happens, gently bring yourself back to your focus. As you continue to practice, being in focus will come with greater ease.

Sometimes it may feel as if you cannot relax your mind, or keep it focused. This is all right because being aware of your tense mind is part of being mindful. Stay present with your mind, and when your thoughts wander, gently bring them back to your focus. Allowing your breathing to slow down will help your mind to slow down too, a little bit at a time.

Returning to everyday life

As you re-enter everyday life, let the wisdom, calm, insight, humour, compassion and spaciousness you gained in meditation filter into your day. Be completely aware of your actions; be present in the moment.

The true miracle of practicing meditation is ordinary and practical. It is a subtle transformation of your mind, body, and soul.

Inspire yourself to meditate with candles, incense, artwork that lifts your spirits, music that feeds your soul, dew on a flower petal, sunlight through the trees, a clear blue sky, and rich velvet. Try different approaches. Slowly you will become master of your own bliss with a collection of remedies that will delight, inspire, illuminate, and elevate your every breath and moment.

Just because you meditate doesn't mean you won't be running around, or that you will be calm all the time. It means that you'll be more aware and present because you stopped for a while to listen, to pause, to watch, and to understand.

10. Communicating mindfully with others

Listening, speaking, watching, feeling how attentive are you when communicating with others? Are you kind, respectful and thoughtful? Do you assume that others automatically understand what you intend to communicate?

It is your responsibility to communicate clearly and, in turn, attend carefully to communication addressed to you. Give others the attention you would like to receive.

> **Often it is our preoccupation with**
> **expressing our own ideas that leaves**
> **us less responsive to others.**

An important aspect of communication is not only what we express, but how we express it. While at some level we understand the difference between inspirational and positive language and words that hurt, control, or denigrate, we don't always put that knowledge into practice.

Over the past few years, while instructing teachers on perception skills I have noted the many long faces showing shocked recognition of how often they inadvertently discouraged children, suppressed creativity, and even dampened their developmental success by unskillful, judgmental language, and perhaps even by words intended as jokes. Adults, too, can be hurt by words hurled with little thought.

Diligent awareness will help you make positive adjustments to your ways of communication, not just in the words you use, but also in body language, general mannerisms and, perhaps most of all, in your ability to listen.

Respectful language habits are critical in developing self-esteem and self-respect, and will eventually influence others to consider how they are communicating. Learning, sharing, encouraging, and negotiating conflict resolution are then workable, accessible, and flowing — to everyone's benefit.

Words that discourage

We are well meaning in our intentions to compliment, praise, and joke. Yet some words and phrases can be so final, relentless, and unforgiving that they are discouraging and demoralizing. Jokes are really not funny when they demean someone else. Nor are harsh tones or sarcasm constructive or motivating.

Sometimes in self-talk we can set ourselves up for failure or disappointment by using competitive and evaluative terms. Some of these are judgment-type words that put us in a category.

Words that tend to label, measure, evaluate, or command may be misconstrued as judgmental, limiting, controlling, or even condemning. For example:

always	*guilt*
never	*if only*
impossible	*supposed to*
have to	*ought to*
should	*however*
can't	*doubt*
must	*but*
regret	*difficult*

Words that inspire competition could be potential set-ups for failure, depending on the connotation and situation:

good	*best*
bad	*great*
better	

Words that instill frustration or fear of failure require careful consideration, especially where there are no absolutes, such as in artistic performance and creativity:

complicated	*wrong*
difficult	*incorrect*
right	*error*
correct	*cheat*
accurate	*unacceptable*
mistake	*hard*

Take a moment to think about the pressure these words can place on someone. To introduce a subject as 'easy' or 'difficult' assumes a value judgment that might not be shared. Consider, instead, whose standard is being presented. Introducing a subject as 'new' or 'fascinating' is more approachable and inspires curiosity. Because of differing abilities, some tasks take varying effort and time. Individuality needs to be accounted for.

Words that encourage

How can you be encouraging? How can you guide, develop, enhance? These questions are not just for teachers in a classroom, but apply to all our relationships:

Acknowledge the validity of someone's statement and his or her right to say it.

Be aware of your words and their impact.

Be aware of your tone.

Respond and praise sincerely; encourage while offering guidance.

Sometimes, explaining your viewpoint and choice of words can soften necessary criticism or correction. Take care to use words appropriately. Here are some suggestions on building words and comments:

In taking responsibility, use 'I' statements for opinions and feelings.

When talking about personal tasks and opinions, appreciate differences and uniqueness without the necessity of agreement or disagreement. Acknowledging the other does not mean you are agreeing.

Think about it. Try it. Here are a few examples.

I like the way you are working.

I am curious...

That's an interesting way of looking at it.

You have figured that out!

Make a list of your own examples.

The external critic

It's wonderful when people believe in you and your greatness. It's even more potent when you believe in yourself.

True encouragement comes gently and builds esteem. Suggestive comments could prompt defensiveness. When you can acknowledge your success and growth to please yourself, then you have the most power because this power emanates from you.

More than language

Various words and meanings can be unclear in any language. Consider the words you use with care. Be open to clarifying, redefining and reconsidering them.

Consider the framework from which you speak: You are using words from your experience, which may not be the same in another culture or situation.

Articulation can be challenging, regardless of how big your vocabulary is, as words alone can be limiting. Tone, body language, and facial expressions add dimension to what is communicated.

Framing, introducing, offering, and being curious are gentle ways to approach communication. Set an intention to be caring and approachable.

11. Active listening

Active or 'experiential' listening is a supportive and non-interfering way of stating back to the speaker what he or she is communicating to you. This enables the speaker to hear what the listener heard. The speaker's message might not be quite what the listener heard.

Language has limitations in meaning and interpretation. What is said is relative to the individual's experience and culture. We hear and speak through the lens of our experience. Framing and introducing ideas set up open communication and curiosity on both sides.

With words and impressions aired on both sides, wrong impressions can be corrected and ideas fleshed out in detail, with a good chance of mutual understanding. Active listening helps people articulate their inner thoughts and processes, and explore ideas and issues. Active listening also gives the speaker an opportunity to hear and understand her- or himself when thoughts are reflected back.

With active listening, repetitive thoughts and beliefs can be lifted out of limbo and brought toward clarity and understanding. We can then use experience and memory to transcend our old ways and contribute fresh thoughts and ideas.

How active listening works

Sometimes one speaker might want to talk through an entire issue before hearing a response from the listener, or the speaker might want to deal with one thought at a time. It helps to agree on a time limit beforehand, and then place an unobtrusive clock nearby. From my experience, we usually can intuitively regulate our attention without feeling that time is a restraint. Usually, the exercise is completed within five minutes of the pre-set time.

For the listener, active participation is more than repeating words. It involves communicating back to the speaker the thoughts, expressions, tone, and even the body language that has been related.

With practice, what at first may seem awkward and laborious can become a natural way of communication.

It is amazing how clear and uncluttered understanding becomes with the effort to listen intently. The energy saved on guesses and assumptions is liberating on both sides.

12. Tuning into music and sound

In ancient cultures, the loudest sounds people heard might be a rumble of thunder or a warrior's battle cry. Since then, the world has become far noisier. There is so much sound and vibration in our lives. Noise from computers, heaters, lights, motors, fans, air conditioners, filters, radios, generators, dryers, machinery, traffic, and more constantly batter us.

Awareness of the importance of sound in your life may be an important beginning for you.

When we learn to tune out some of the noise, we may also be tuning out sounds that could be important. How do we select and how do we edit? Do some sounds get filed in the 'ignore' pile and others not? What messages need to be heard? Perhaps we don't even know. Who knows what we are missing?

How can we appreciate sound if we don't listen? How can we listen if we don't appreciate sound?

As we block noise, are we also learning to block other senses and other sensations? Are we numbing ourselves to the world around us? No wonder that we're exhausted at the end of the day. We crave greenery and rivers and quiet.

Check your environment throughout your day. Can some sounds be turned down? Can sound-emitting machines be moved or muffled? Can your work area be shifted to a quieter location? What can we control?

Try to take breaks from the cacophony of daily noise.

Turn off the TV. Turn down the radio. Find a quiet area to read in or just to reflect. Spend time in a visual or aural sanctuary like a forest, a garden, or a park. If that's not possible, develop images in your mind of quiet, restful spaces, and now and then tune out the noise and just visualize those places. Think of the silence of underwater scuba diving, the gentle slapping of water against a canoe. Imagine yourself in a comfy wicker chair on a sunny porch. If outside noise prevents this, use headphones and nature tapes until you can do it in a natural environment.

Sometimes, turn everything off and just sit quietly. Pull up those calm, silent visions.

Listen to the sound of silence and feel yourself relaxing.

Music is associated with creation

The ancient world knew the miraculous power of music for harmonizing body and spirit.

Many cultures still use various sounds to inspire healing, for spiritual enlightenment, and for tuning into the energy of the universe. Music is a universal language and anyone can benefit from its uplifting powers. It has no barriers of prejudice or location.

Musical vibrations can stimulate everything. If it is true that plants grow best near calming music, then surely calming music is good for humans, too.

✦   Select music to enhance your life.

✦   Listen and note how various kinds of music make you feel.

✦   Which style relaxes you?

✦   If you want to rev up, what type of music does that for you?

I use music in my workshops as background or sometimes as a focusing tool. Participants comment on their relaxation level and their successes. Observers notice increased calm and concentration in the students. The few times when I have left music out, my students tell me they miss it.

For workshops, I try to pick music that blends into the background. Music can relax and mellow a classroom or liven it up.

Music can evoke powerful emotions and unlock either happy or sad experiences stored in our memories. Combining music with imagery and other art forms intensifies and expands the experience

Gaining a deeper awareness of sounds can help you to understand how sound affects you.

Explore different ways of experiencing sound. Use colours, shapes, and journaling to give expression to the sounds you hear.

Consider different musical instruments, such as a drum, shakers, violin, piano, flute, and so on, and try to understand how each affects you. Are the sounds soothing, irritating, inspiring, heartfelt, sad...?

Also collect musical recordings that use instruments in different ways, and from different cultures. For example, for drumming try East Indian, African, North American First Nations, Chilean, and jazz kit drumming. Option: listen and explore your response to sounds of daily living; for example, a blender, a ringing phone, a boiling kettle, or water dripping.

Rhythm and vibration

Exploring different rhythms is something that we feel with our whole body. When the music is right for us, we want to yield to it and move with its rhythms and vibrations. We feel motivated, relaxed, and rejuvenated.

Scientifically speaking, we are energy vibrating at a cellular level. All other matter is vibrating, too. Since vibrations are rhythms, everything is rhythm. All vibrations interconnect and interact with each other.

**Life is challenging enough without
going against the natural rhythms
of the world around us.**

In nature, it takes less energy to pulse together than to pulse in opposition, so similar rhythms tend to align over time. Becoming aware of the signals within our bodies helps us align with and communicate with other rhythms. As you explore rhythm, you tap into collective energy. It is indescribable. Experiencing it is the only way.

+ Body rhythms and patterns. We are all musical. We are born with body rhythms and patterns. Our bodies are rhythm machines, in and out of sync, creating patterns and chaos. Our heartbeat is the most familiar. In First Nations traditions, it is said that, when we drum, we are echoing our heartbeat for the earth.

+ Listen.

+ Listen more.

+ Respond.

When exploring different rhythms, relax and let your whole being feel and move to the vibrations. You will know in your body and in your mind and with all your senses the rightness of what rhythms resonate with your rhythm. You will feel it in your hands and in your feet, and you will want to give in to the rhythm. Dare to let yourself go.

Dancing with passion

Dance ugliness, dance anger, and dance wildly. Sweat. Even if you hate the music, give in to it! Dance as if you hate it! Respond to it! Dance fearful!

Dance is about passion. Dance dreamily, softly, gracefully, and exotically.

Dance anywhere. Dance with life as your lover.

Dance gleeful! For no other reason except for glee itself, jump! Do a cool move. Do an awkward move. Tell a story in your dance.

The body needs to move and to dance. Sing and hum to your own rhythm and timing.

Drumming, dancing, chanting, singing, and humming are ways to infiltrate other vibrations into your cells. As you practise awareness of your rhythm, you will be able to further relate to other rhythms around you. These rhythms of humanity, the weather, earth cycles like seasons and tides, society, and systems are everywhere. With your regained sensitivity, you will be able to adjust yourself and resonate with similar rhythms, thus gaining some harmony with your surroundings.

13. Managing food intolerance

While food is essential for our survival, some foods may work against us, making us feel anxious.

+ The food intolerance test is a food test you can order and pay for privately with a referral from your family doctor. The test checks for foods your body proteins may have trouble breaking down and utilizing, and produces a chart indicating those foods to which your body is intolerant, or borderline intolerant. The test rates more than 200 foods.

+ It is different from a food allergy test. Being allergic to foods may mean that your body has an anaphylactic rapid onset of symptoms after consuming a particular food.

+ Digesting food your body cannot tolerate may not produce clear symptoms. Eating foods that you are intolerant to could exacerbate irritable bowel syndrome, and cause such symptoms as bloating, anxiety, headaches, fatigue, asthma, joint pain, arthritis, weight problems, fibromyalgia, and itchy skin.

Many people have taken both food intolerance and allergy tests, and as a result were able to eliminate troublesome foods. I have had several clients take this test with great results. Removing some foods has helped children with behaviour and sleep issues. It has helped adults with Irritable Bowel Syndrome (IBS) and improved their moods. One of my clients reported the complete absence of headaches after taking the test and making appropriate dietary changes.

I recently took the test and was surprised about some of the foods on my food intolerance list, such as white beans, peas, and almonds. However, I am eliminating them to increase my resilience and health. Since the test I have kept a short diary and have noticed mood changes based on eating foods that I have lower tolerance for. At this moment I can say that when I avoid foods on my intolerance list, I seem to feel more resilient and calmer.

14. Replenishing your diet

Learning how and what to eat has become an education industry in itself. From the perspective of managing stress and anxiety, here are a few essentials.

Magnesium

Magnesium is a valuable resource that many of my client-parents have used for their children to help lower their anxiety and help them sleep.

Magnesium is known as a vital enzyme catalyst, especially of those enzymes involved in energy production. It also helps the body absorb calcium and potassium.

A deficiency in magnesium interferes with the transmission of nerve and muscle impulses, causing irritability and nervousness. Having enough magnesium can help prevent depression, dizziness, muscle weakness and twitching, and pre-menstrual syndrome. It also helps the body maintain proper pH levels and normal body temperature.

Magnesium is an essential mineral and does a lot in the body. It occurs naturally in many food sources: fish, meat, seafood, apples, apricots, avocados, bananas, and blackstrap molasses, to name a few.

I won't go through all the benefits here. If you are interested in learning more, see the references in the back of the book.

Calcium

It is commonly known that calcium can have a calming effect on the nervous system. When the body is low on calcium, nerve cells can go into hyperactivity. Magnesium and calcium balance each other and work well together. If you have concerns about lack of minerals in your body, consult a health practitioner. Also, turn to the references in the back of the book for more information.

Other calming resources

Magnesium and calcium are just two of many natural dietary resources. Vitamin supplements such as Vitamin B-complex and Vitamin C help increase your resilience to stress.

Bach Therapy, also called Flower Remedies: This method of treatment, and its 38 remedies, was developed by Edward Bach, a well-known physician in the 1930s. The remedies, still widely used today, are all prepared from flowers, plants, bushes, and trees. None of them is harmful or habit forming. I have used Bach Rescue Remedy for myself and brought up my children with it. I carry it in my purse and have it by my bedside table. Rescue Remedy contains five of the Bach flower remedies.

Herbs and herbal teas such as chamomile, peppermint, and holy basil are some of the calming teas.

Although aromatherapy and essential oils are definitely not a dietary resource, I include them here because they're from natural sources and serve as food for the soul. Specifically for relaxing, I enjoy using lavender and many other essential oils.

15. Protecting yourself

We tend to associate empowering ourselves with taking action. Sometimes the process requires a restorative or protective pause before we wade back into the stream of things. Here are three ways your inner warrior can protect you.

Protector/shield

A few years ago, I went to a meeting and came home wiped out, tired, and depressed. It had been a good day, but I felt terrible. I remember going to my tai chi class and my instructor said I was too open. I said

I thought we were to be open? "No," she said. "Imagine yourself as a lotus flower. Sometimes the blossom opens itself entirely to the world, but at other times the blossom closes itself a little or even a lot, protecting itself from negative and unhealthy experiences." This was my first introduction to the concept of shielding myself.

The goal is to create/imagine a shield that can be used anytime and anywhere. This is especially useful for people who are highly sensitive and empathic. For instance, someone who, while sitting beside a sad person, also begins to feel sad.

Imagine your own shield, one that could protect you. This shield can be a knight's shield, a warrior, a row of flowers, a waterfall, a curtain, or a bulletproof bubble. My shield protects me. One client uses a circle of skunks. Sometimes, getting dressed can be a metaphor for a shield, or wearing certain jewelry or stones can symbolize the protection.

Another client, a young child, was being bullied at school. He was a chess prodigy, and to shield himself imagined his adversaries as queens. I asked him, "Doesn't the queen have a lot of power in chess?" He said with a smile, "Yeah, but they're girls." After that the bullying no longer bothered him and it eventually stopped.

Do what works for you. Find a quiet spot, notice your breathing, take time to imagine your shield, notice its qualities, and how your body feels.

This shield protects and keeps you safe. It keeps out others' unpleasant moods, gossip, verbal bullying, another's business, the irritation of bad drivers, and so on. You can still be empathic and remain aware, but most of the unpleasantness stays on the outside.

I use the shield in my work. If I did not protect my sensitive nature, I would not be able to work with trauma clients.

You can even use it to go shopping — who knows what type of energy or unskillfulness will appear?

Just because you install a shield once, doesn't mean you will never be caught off guard. However, installing it regularly and reinforcing it makes the skill stronger. I install my shield before I get out of bed in the morning, and I reinforce it all day long.

Here is another wonderful concept to include as part of your shield. Byron Katie uses this. It is called 'god's business, your business, my business'. (Bari McFarland also refers to this in her chapter; see page 118).

We have no control over the business of god (the God of your understanding; Spirit/Mother Nature, Yahweh, and so on). It is the weather, acts of nature, the way a flower blooms, and so on. There is really no sense in getting wrapped up in it in a negative way, as there is nothing we can do about it.

Your business: your business is really none of my business. So, if you are making poor choices, that is your business. If you are regularly negative and have a negative attitude, that is your business. If you have not asked me for my help, that is your business. Your thoughts are your business.

My business is what goes on between my ears. My business is my choice on how to think, what to think, how to imagine, and how to act. My thoughts are my business.

I can leave your business outside my shield. I can notice, though I need not get wrapped up in it, interfere in it, take it on or let it into my personal sphere.

Container

Using a container in the mind is another great strategy in mind control. Sometimes we have unpleasant memories or feelings. Sometimes these unpleasant feelings are invasive. Often we have learned to push away these unpleasant feelings, or stuff them away. This only increases the pain. And when this builds up, it clouds all emotions. Eventually, we have difficulty discerning whether we are feeling happy, sad, angry, and so on. These feelings can also build up to the extent that a) we get tired of suppressing them, and b) it does not take much to tip us over the edge, into depression or anger.

The container is a way of putting unpleasant memories and emotions away. It involves acknowledging them, which is different from stuffing them away. They get to stay, safely contained, until you want to deal with them, process them, and/or heal them.

Imagine a container, any container. Some people have several containers. This container has the ability to hold whatever you want to put in it. Make sure that you can lock it and store it somewhere safe.

Take your time and put anything you want to put in this container for safe and secure holding.

Sometimes, the feelings or memories may ooze out. Just put them back in and lock them up. After some practice they usually stay put. The difference between storing things in this container versus pushing them away or suppressing them is that we are conscious of what we are storing away.

Safe/calm place

I have used many versions of this exercise. It is another grounding exercise, and is especially effective when having higher levels of anxiety.

Imagine a place of well-being, calm, peace, and stillness. This place can be real or imaginary. This place could be a holiday, a place in nature, a family cottage, a sacred place, a grandmother's kitchen, a sanctuary. It could be inside your heart. This place has many positive feelings, memories, and sensations.

Imagine yourself there, the sights, the sounds, any smells. Notice how your body feels when you are there. Do you feel, settled, cozy, comfortable? What is your breathing like, has it slowed down? What emotions do you feel — comfort, ease, settled, happy, at peace, joyful, cared for?

'Calm place' is a wonderful exercise to get children to settle down at night or during the day when they are feeling anxious.

16. Journaling, and journaling ideas

Writing is known as one of the cleansing and healing tools of the mind. Writing uses the mind's tools of language and images to express thoughts and feelings, either factually or imaginatively.

Sometimes our thoughts are buried behind judgments, low self-esteem, personal doubt and/or concern about the opinions of others. Journal writing is private and personal, and it's intended only for you. The act of writing random thoughts and describing ideas and images can release us from tension and put us on the threshold of exciting creativity.

Journal writing can be your private and unique act of expression without concern for form, style, grammar, or even punctuation.

Writing also often provides the raw material for creating art. As with other art forms such as song writing, painting, and poetry, we often belittle our own ability to create. We often carry strong judgments on how art in any form should be expressed. We think that we aren't smart enough, original enough, or travelled enough.

Journaling can be wondrous

Thoughts have a tendency to mill around in our minds. It often seems that the mind, when cluttered with unacknowledged thoughts, has little space to play with new ideas and creative possibilities. However, when writing down your thoughts, something transcendental happens. The act of writing them down seems to acknowledge their existence, and permits you to move on. This creates more room for fresh thought and new ideas. These written-down thoughts become 'something' outside yourself. One can look at these thoughts outside one's self, consider them and/or turn the page.

Make room at the beginning of your day to sit for a few minutes and become quietly aware of your thoughts. Notice them throughout the day. You may soon become aware of how many thoughts keep repeating. By writing them down as they spin through your mind, you will slow them down. When these thoughts are acknowledged and put on the shelf, it leaves space for the new thoughts. As you check in with yourself you will learn about yourself.

Regular journaling helps houseclean your mind, keeping it fresh, clear, and open for constructive and creative thoughts. It also provides a record of past ideas and concerns, and can make you aware of the value of language and words.

Journaling ideas

Your journal is personal, private, and confidential. Perhaps it is a daily check-in? Perhaps a dumping ground? Perhaps it will hold memories or reasons for gratitude? Maybe sketches? And/or a workbook for poetry?

Don't criticize your writing or your drawing. Do what feels right for you. Trust yourself to know what you need and follow your own impulses. Enjoy your road to discovery.

Here are 26 ideas that might help you get started.

1. How do I feel about myself today?

2. Did I comfort myself in any way?

3. Did I punish myself in any way?

4. How did other people treat me today, what did I do, and

how did I respond? Was I more concerned about pleasing others than in meeting my own needs? Did anyone say anything that sticks in my mind or that seemed to have some special meaning or importance to me?

5. Did I observe anything or did I do anything that left an impression on me?

6. If I were to live this day over, how would I change it and why?

7. My hopes and dreams are...

8. In the future I want...

9. I wonder about...

10. What puzzles me is...

11. I am unsure about...

12. What's interesting is...

13. What's hard about this is...

14. One place I will grow is...

15. A strength for me is...

16. Something I am noticing is...

17. I'm surprised at...

18. I learned...

19. I am concerned that...

20. This is different because...

21. I feel connected...

22. It made me think about...

23. I could visualize...

24. I figured out...

25. I can relate this to...

26. When do I notice my body energy rising? And when do I notice my body energy dropping?

Give it a try now. Notice how your body and mood change? (See *Creative Practices*, number 15, page 146, 'Journaling'.)

17. Journaling your gratitude

> **"It is not joy that makes us grateful; it is gratitude that makes us joyful."**
> — *Brother David Steindl-Rast*

Practising gratitude is one of the quickest ways to change your mindset.

The key word is 'practising'. I have been practising gratitude in my journal morning and night daily for over eight years. My attitude and mind have changed and I choose to live and begin each day with a joyful heart. It is a 'practice' as well. Some days I may not feel grateful. However, by the time I am done my practice I feel good.

For me this practice started with a question: How was I going to make the 'joy property' bigger than the 'trauma property' in my brain?

A few years ago, upon waking up and before going to sleep, I would mentally list things I was grateful for, though many times I was distracted and did not get very far, or I would forget. A wise counsellor had me recount positive stories and experiences to him. He suggested repeating these stories in my mind over and over again, and to share them with others. I could also put 'props' up to remind me of those wonderful times. How could I use this idea, I wondered, to make the gratitude feeling deeper and bigger?

I had heard that Tibetan monks bring an empty bowl to their morning meditation, trusting that the bowl will be filled by the end of the day with the things that they need. No matter how the day goes, something always gets put in the bowl. I put an empty bowl in my bedroom and it is now one of the first things I see when I open my eyes. This practice has helped make the happier memories bigger in my brain.

I did begin to experience joy on occasion, though I generally still felt somewhat flat. Even though I still knew how tremendously lucky

I was (and am), that bubbling joy still hid from me.

To further the list of things I'm grateful for, I began a small gratitude journal. It was a very tiny journal. My belief is that if it is small, and if it takes little effort, then I am more likely to do it.

So every morning upon waking, I would fill a tiny page with things I was grateful for. This progressed to morning and night time.

After about a year, I wondered how I could expand my positive experience of gratitude and joy to ripple throughout the day. I progressed to larger journals! I began pausing as I was writing my gratitude list, letting the experience of what I was writing have a few more moments. I also began doodling little hearts and exclamation marks on the tiny pages. I pasted inspirational sayings into my journal. I would look back at written pages and smile at events or listed items and remember them happening.

I noticed that a feeling of deep love and gratitude permeated my whole body. At first, it took me by surprise. A joyful, excited feeling was dancing in my body. Then I realized I was finally expanding my inner joy to a point of inner dancing and ecstasy.

Try gratitude journaling for yourself. See *Creative Practices*, number 16 (page 147).

18. Worrying assignment

We are more than our brains. Our brains function on the history of memory and experience.

Our brains are often cluttered with random thoughts. Be aware of repetitive, negative, and unyielding mind chatter.

Some negative thoughts include all-or-nothing thinking, black-and-white thinking, jumping to conclusions, or making rash assumptions. Sometimes past problems, such as situations taken personally, and blaming yourself or others inappropriately can crowd out positive reflections. Negative thoughts can make us overlook the roles and responsibilities of others, or cause us to fail to consider the whole picture.

Take charge of your thoughts. Be aware of uncompromising mind chatter and edit it accordingly. It takes practice to do this, so be patient with yourself. Notice when your inner critic is attacking you. Does it seem to happen most often when you are tired? Hungry? Are the thoughts a habit? Does it occur in the company of certain people?

What are your triggers? Often, such thoughts gang up on you when you have excluded the positive elements in your life by focusing on what was lost, instead of what is available.

Try looking at each situation differently. Reword your thinking. Walith practice, you will quickly identify mind comments that are not serving you and you can quickly delete them. Be easy on yourself, because some of these thought patterns and 'mind tapes' may be embedded and resist your attempts to evict them. Gradually, through your awareness of their negativity, you will be able to identify self-defeating mind ramblings and 'set them on a shelf', or delete them.

Making yourself aware of negative thoughts makes it possible for you to edit them accordingly.

Scheduling your drama and worry time

Long ago a good friend of mine, Bess Jones, suggested that negative, unproductive issues deserve some attention. Instead of worrying off and on all day long, she said to allot only 10 to 20 minutes to wallow in the depths of worry and drama.

When I first tried giving in to those 'down' feelings — but only for a set time — I used a timer. However, I rarely needed the full time. I learned that permitting oneself to deliberately focus on those feelings, rather than fighting them, bores the brain.

Try to rewrite thoughts in a positive way. For example: replace "I always waste time" with "I can best spend time by…" When the time invested in worry or despair is adequate, the brain is able to move on and experience what the rest of the day has to offer.

Worrying can be very helpful if it means looking at a problem from different sides and developing a solution. However, worrying can be unhelpful if your thoughts go around and around and you can't stop. It becomes an activity that takes a lot of energy.

In these instances a 'worrying assignment' can be helpful. This assignment is meant to make worrying fruitful again. Real worrying can play an important role in helping us become aware of problems and solutions.

Worrying assignment

It is best if you work on this assignment half an hour per day and start worrying deliberately. Find a quiet spot where you can write undisturbed. Take a pen and paper, and write down everything that comes to mind. Write all your worries over and over again for the full allotted time. Try, if possible, to write at the same time each day.

You will notice that, by the conscious and concentrated effort of the worrying sessions, it becomes almost impossible to continue thinking in circles. This is reinforced by writing. Usually, nobody writes down the same thoughts 12 times. This forces the thoughts to go in different directions.

In addition to this, thoughts that are written down encourage fleshing out the problems.

You will notice that this assignment restores the original goal of worrying, meaning that outside of the worrying sessions, it will become easier to let go of fruitless worrying. If your brain begins to worry again after the finishing the worry assignment, pause and let your brain know that it can worry in the next allotted time. And then think about something else. Clients report that their thoughts change and they have either solved their problems or that they rarely worry.

19. How to introduce new habits

As I was growing personally and professionally, I heard that building a new habit variously takes 21 days, 33 days, a month, and so on. I was rarely successful when I used these time frames. John Gray's book, *Venus and Mars in the Bedroom*, states that the brain needs to hear a concept at least 200 times to accept it; 150 times if you are a genius.

This fascinated me and lead me to researching more about creating new habits.

Phillippa Lally is a health psychology researcher at University College London. In a study published in the European Journal of Social Psychology,[1] Lally and her research team decided to figure out just how long forming a habit actually takes.

The study examined the habits of 96 people over a 12-week period. Each person chose one new habit for the 12 weeks and reported each day on whether or not they performed the behaviour and how automatic it felt.

Some people chose simple habits like drinking a bottle of water with lunch. Others chose more difficult tasks like running for 15 minutes before dinner. At the end of 12 weeks, the researchers analysed the data to determine how long it had taken each person to go from starting a new behaviour to automatically doing it.

The answer? On average, it takes more than two months, or 66 days, before a new behaviour becomes automatic. How long it takes a new habit to form can vary widely depending on the new behaviour, the person, and the circumstances. In Lally's study, it took anywhere from 18 days to 254 days for people to form a new habit.

In other words, if you want to set your expectations appropriately, the truth is that it will probably take you anywhere from two months to eight months to build a new behaviour into your life, not 21 days.

Interestingly, the researchers also found that "missing one opportunity to perform the behaviour did not materially affect the habit formation process." In other words, it doesn't matter if you mess up every now and then. Building better habits is not an all-or-nothing process.

This study is encouraging.

As you continue through this book, you'll encounter some brilliant contributors. These authors are writers, presenters, teachers, and facilitators. They are passionate about their topics and live them. Since this is what they do in their lives, I invited them to share. In the event a chapter resonates with you, you'll find the author's biography and contact information at the end of the book.

Note

1 Phillippa Lally, Cornelia H. M. van Jaarsveld, Henry W. W. Potts, Jane Wardle, "How are habits formed: Modelling habit formation in the real world," European Journal of Social Psychology, July 16, 2009; http://onlinelibrary.wiley.com/doi/10.1002/ejsp.674/abstract.

Financial Anxiety

by Ryan Brown

As a single mother I struggled with poverty, although I did not fully grasp the 'poverty' label. I always felt and still feel lucky. I learned to maximize a dollar, making it count as if it were 10 dollars. In my early 20s I met a unique bank manager who taught me marketing, budgeting, planning, and researching. He opened me to the possibilities and made it clear that I was the customer and he valued my business. 'Kel' was not a typical bank manager or lender. Because of him, I set financial goals and researched how I could achieve them creatively. Ryan Brown reminds me of Kel. Ryan is passionate about empowering people financially, he sees simple ways to do this, and believes we can do it.

Worrying about our finances can undermine our health, threaten our relationships, and lead us to question our self-worth. It can perpetuate itself, demoralizing us to the point where we don't see any way out. It undermines the very foundation of our 'Maslow', a universal hierarchy of personal needs. Mastering these needs allows us to live life fully and become the best we can.[1]

I know this from my own experience years ago, and from my private therapy practice today, where financial anxiety is a constant topic of discussion.

Helping people manage their financial anxiety is also a priority for Ryan, who encounters it from another perspective. Ryan is a debt relief specialist with a Canadian company named 4 Pillars Consulting Group, and has made it his life's work to help people get out from under the debt that causes them such crushing anxiety.

In a wide-ranging conversation, Ryan shared with me his perspective on financial anxiety, as well as essential advice on how to regain control of your financial situation. Here are some of the highlights.

— Elke

Ryan, why do you do this kind of work?

It started when I was working with businesses to help them improve cash flow and grow. It was during this time that I learned about how interest rate changes and carrying debt to operate your business could very quickly shut the doors on your business.

The more involved I became, the more I realized it wasn't about numbers on a page, but the effect debt could have on people. When someone is overwhelmed with debt, they sleep with it, they go to work with it... Debt can stop us from doing the things we enjoy, or enjoying the things we're doing. In so many cases it stops us from growing as a person and doing better in our careers.

I also saw the effect debt relief could have. I've worked with a couple who, on their first visit, sat on opposite sides from each other. After a couple of meetings, they were sitting together. Their whole demeanor changed. I've also seen people who, once their financial burden has been lifted, perform better at work, earning raises and promotions because they're no longer distracted by their debt situation.

I remember you telling me about a client you didn't recognize from one visit to the next.

A client walked in and I said, "Hi, how are you today? How can I help you?" She said, "Well, I'm here for my appointment, Ryan."

This was only her second appointment, and she looked many years younger. Like a different person. She had realized there were manageable solutions to her financial problems, and she felt relief.

How much debt do we have collectively?

Canadians as a whole are approximately $2 trillion in debt. Yes, this includes mortgages, but a mortgage is one of the most expensive debts anyone could ever take on. I have come across many clients carrying a mortgage on a house that has gone down in value, which is also a risk aside from just carrying the debt.

From 1980 to 2005, Canadians' annual income increased by close to only $50 per annum in constant dollars.[2] Yet the average house price increased well beyond the average inflation rate over the same time frame, by about 400%.[3] So in this situation, servicing a mortgage takes a greater percentage of a person's income, unless of course we extend the terms out to 25, 30, 35 years, which is exactly what many people have done. As a result, people nowadays are generally paying a lot more interest because the term of the mortgage is so long. The only way house prices could go up as they have, is to make them affordable to buy while the price goes up. Again, you do this with no money down and 30-year amortizations.

So in saying all of that, yes we hear that a lot of debt which Canadians carry is mortgage debt and this is supposed to make us feel better. But the fact remains, $2 trillion of debt is $2 trillion of debt, and interest eats away at profits.

Here are a few more statistics. From 1977 to 2011, the population grew by 35%.[4] At the same time, the number of Visa® and Master-Card® credit cards in circulation grew by almost 900%, from 8.2 million to 74.5 million. Spending on those cards rose 8,100%, from $4.04 billion to $331.81 billion.[5]

We have a debt culture. It's become 'normal' for people to accept debt. There's also a belief that we have to have access to credit in case something happens. Sometimes we're not even paying for our own life challenges any more, we may be financing them.

We're seeing a lot of seniors now carrying debt into retirement. Everywhere we go, we're marketed to consume stuff. What happened to the days of being content and enjoying the moment? Gone.

We're the saddest, most depressed continent on the planet. Materially we have the most, but we're being told we don't have enough.

It doesn't have to be this way. There are simple things we can do to manage our debt and our financial anxiety. It's not necessarily about going out and making more money.

How much of this is due to lack of financial awareness?

We hear a lot about financial literacy and IQ. Honestly, it's not rocket science. Sometimes it comes down to people not being content. Everywhere we go, we're encouraged to spend. Why does everyone believe they have to own a house? For most of us, having a house means having a mortgage. My parents didn't have a house until I was in Grade 3. Now I see newly-marrieds buying 3,000 to 4,000 square foot houses. We're all encouraged to overbuy. This is how we get into trouble.

But it's not always about spending habits. I have seen what seems to be an endless number of hardship cases. Health challenges, medical costs, debilitating injuries, inheritances causing financial challenges, unamicable divorces, and the list goes on. So it is not always about spending habits. In saying all of that, in every case proper financial planning early in life, be that proper insurances, savings plans, living on less, etc., could provide some help when financial challenges arise.

Eleven ways to reduce your debt and free yourself from financial anxiety

Taking that first step to regain control of your finances is never easy, but the potential mental health benefits are immense. In our conversation, Ryan offered a number of methods we can use to regain control of our financial health. What works best for you depends on your particular circumstances.

If you feel overwhelmed by your financial situation, talk to an expert like Ryan. But first, start with Ryan's sample suggestions, as follows:

1. **Be honest with yourself.** What's the root cause of your indebtedness? Many people who come to me have got into debt because of health issues that prevent them from working, they've lost their job, they're divorced... Some people are dealing with multiple factors. Is the debt the main problem, or a symptom of an underlying problem? If you don't recognize the challenges, you can't identify solutions.

2. **Understand what you spend your money on.** Some people don't want to know because they're afraid of what they'll see, but if we don't keep track, we'll never know. It's all right there in your bank statements. Once you know where your money is going, you can control the flow. I know this from personal experience. At one point in my life I was driving 1,000 kilometres per week to meet with clients. I came home one night and my wife asked me if I knew how much money I had spent the previous month while on the road. I had no idea, so I figured it out: $900. Then I had to ask myself what that $900 had got me. Nothing but a backseat full of empty coffee cups. Remember, spending rises to meet income. For many of us, as we make more money, we don't always end up with more money.

3. **Don't be afraid of dealing with debt.** Don't let your anxiety prevent you from taking that important first step. I have seen it way too often, where people have struggled for years with debt before finally contacting us. That adds up to a lot of anxiety, as well as money and time wasted. Dealing with debt can be a smooth, clean process, and with the right tools and the right people supporting you, you may find solutions that can keep you free from financial anxiety for the rest of your life, and that's a big deal. But I cannot stress enough the importance of working with someone who has your best interests in mind. Working with someone who represents your creditors or a company that takes funding from your creditors may not make the most sense.

    You want to find a local person or company that will work with and for you. One that has a long history of success with their clients. You don't want to risk filing an insolvency that wipes you out financially for years to come. I have seen people get into consumer proposals — a legal agreement between you and your creditors to repay part of the debt that you owe — which they cannot afford, and struggle financially for years just to make the payments. Or worse, who then end up still filing bankruptcy after a couple of years because they cannot afford their proposal. The entire process might take 10 years before it clears their credit bureau. If you ask me, that doesn't sound like relief. None of my clients has ever had to come back to me for help with debt. That's a good thing.

4. **Understand your options.** While your debt may feel overwhelming, bankruptcy or a consumer proposal isn't necessarily the answer. With the right support, you can put in place a realistic and achievable debt reduction plan. In saying that, a consumer proposal done with the clients' best interests and future goals in mind is quite possibly the best way to aggressively solve debt in Canada. I say "with the clients' best interests in mind" because the majority of the companies out there who claim to help people solve debt are either a) taking funding from the creditors or b) representing the creditors. Most people seeking debt help are not privy to this little known yet all important fact.

5. **Create a cash flow management plan.** People often think
   this means, "You're going to tell me how to spend my
   money," or "You're going to tell me what to do without."
   What I'm really going to tell them is how they can save
   their money. I understand the fear, but putting together
   and following a budget can actually free you from fear. In
   my case, after that conversation with my wife, I created a
   very simple plan that tracked expenses daily. Each evening
   I would spend five minutes looking at my bank account
   online, recording what I had spent that day, and comparing
   it to my receipts. It quickly became a regular habit. In place
   of fear, I had a new understanding of where my money was
   going, and was able to make informed choices about where
   I wanted it to go.

6. **Manage your finances like a business.** Take your utility bill as an example. Every January my wife and I would
   receive a $900-1000 electric utility bill, right after Christ-
   mas. It used to drive me nuts. If you're self employed, you
   may barely be making money during the two weeks around
   Christmas. My wife and I called the utility, which offered
   to equalize our billing. "Sure," they said. "It will be $300/
   month." We weren't satisfied with that, because the utility
   would be collecting more than we owed. "Well, there will be
   a credit there for you at the end of the year," they explained.
   But my wife and I were not interested in overpaying as we
   were looking to manage cash flow. We decided instead to
   equal bill ourselves. We paid that big January bill, looked at
   the last two years' bills, and began to pay $250 per month,
   every month, even when the bill was actually only $100 per
   month. We never saw a $900 bill again, and it felt good.

7. **Pay yourself first.** This is the 10% rule: every time you
   get paid, put 10% into a savings account that isn't easy to
   access. Don't link the account to your debit card, and don't
   tell me you can't afford it. I've seen enough client account
   statements to know you can.

8. **Lower your credit card limit(s) to a reasonable amount.**
   Having excess credit is just an inducement to spend more.
   We live in a consumer culture. If the credit card company

increases your credit limit, ask them to return it to the
previous level.

9. **Avoid day-to-day temptation.** Stop carrying your credit
   and debit cards around with you and (re)learn how to live
   in a cash world. When I was a kid, my dad would come
   home Friday afternoons at lunch and hand my mom an
   envelope with his pay cheque. My mom and I would go to
   the bank, stand in line for a teller, hand them the cheque,
   and have most of it deposited into a bill-paying account,
   a little bit moved into savings, and the rest into cash for
   weekend expenses. If you didn't have it in hand, you didn't
   spend it. This was the early 1980s. There were no bank
   machines, no online banking, and no telephone banking. If
   you didn't have it in your jeans, you weren't spending it.

10. **Ask people you regularly do business with if they have
    any suggestions on how to save money.** They may have
    special offers or promotions you're not aware of. Elke shared
    an example with me. When her monthly shipping bill went
    up significantly, she spent some time going over the bills.
    She realized that if she shipped every two months instead of
    monthly, she'd pay the same fee just once, not twice. Small,
    steady savings like this add up. Imagine the savings over
    five or 10 years.

11. **Be wary of easy solutions.** There are plenty of predatory
    lenders out there. It is my understanding that in Canada,
    interest rates exceeding 60% are considered criminal rates
    of interest. However, I have seen loans in my office that
    have been as high as 127% interest after considering fees
    and other expenses that are tacked on to the purchase price.
    So, just because you are buying from a qualified licensed
    financial institution does not mean you should not read
    and understand what you are signing. Before making any
    decisions, walk away and fully calculate the cost. Keep emo-
    tions out of buying decisions. One time I had a client who
    financed a vehicle purchase. As we were reviewing their
    financial situation, I came across the finance agreement
    for the vehicle. I told the client that they owed $37,000 on
    the vehicle they were driving. They disagreed and insisted

they only owed $20,000. When I showed them one of the last pages of the finance agreement, they were shocked. After their multi-year term of paying for their vehicle, they would still owe what is called a balloon payment of another $17,000. I would not say that this lender was predatory in any way. What I would say is that things were signed very quickly without proper review, as the clients were simply excited to get into their brand new vehicle.

Debt Danger — Know the Warning Signs and Solutions

by Julie Bissonette

I met Julie when she spoke at a local networking meeting. She was encouraging and had a lot to offer.

— Elke

If your debt load is heavier than you want it to be, you are not alone. According to Statistics Canada, Canadian household debt-to-income ratios have reached record highs — ranging above 150%, which means that Canadians owe $1.50 for every dollar of disposable income they have.

Here are a few strategies to help you manage your debt and relieve the anxiety that debt can create.

- ✦ **Take charge of your cards.** A high credit card limit can be a benefit — or a trap — if it influences you to buy more than you can afford. Spending more than you can pay off each month and the interest, often at rates of more than 20%, really builds up on the balance. The key: spend within your means, and pay off your credit card balance each month. You'll avoid debt and take full advantage of any reward points offered by your card(s).

- ✦ **Check your impulses.** That giant TV certainly looks great, but do you really need it? The key: think before you buy. Weigh your options and make prudent purchasing decisions. You'll avoid escalating debt and lingering buyer's remorse.

✦ Protect your credit rating. Be sure the information in your credit report is accurate by checking it at least once a year and reporting any inaccuracies. The two major Canadian credit rating/reporting agencies are Equifax Canada, Inc. (www.equifax.com) and TransUnion Canada (www.transunion.ca). Ensure you pay bills on time and avoid late payments.

✦ **Take command of your life.** Establish a realistic strategy for saving toward your most important life goals. The key: reduce 'bad' debt (credit cards). Explore debt consolidation and a monthly debt reduction plan. Once you work on reducing your debt, then you can start focusing on savings strategies to help you reach your goals. Savings trends have declined over the last 50 years, so it is important to pay yourself first. Put a savings plan in your budget and recognize that the savings plan is just as important a payment as the cell phone bill or the utility bill. It is the only payment in your budget that goes to you and your future. Every other bill you pay goes to someone else and their future.

✦ **Love what you have.** Next time you peer over the fence at the Jones' seemingly greener grass, remind yourself that things don't equal happiness. Remember to prioritize your wants and spend on things that have the most value for you. Make purchases thoughtfully and deliberately, and recognize what factors are influencing your buying decisions. Finally, don't forget about the many things you have to be grateful for and that "comparison is the thief of joy."

Depending on your personal situation, there are other debt reduction and money-saving strategies that could help alleviate stress and get you debt free. Get back on track for financial security. A well thought-out plan for your financial future is an integral part of building the life you want for yourself and your family. As the number of options for investing increase, so does the volume of information available on financial matters. With all this information overload, advice has never been more important.

A financial advisor can provide both a third-party perspective and the financial planning expertise to develop a plan that will work for you. Lightening your debt load, saving more, planning for a financially secure future — a professional advisor can help you get there.

Notes

1 See the *Glossary* for definition of Maslow's hierarchy of needs.
2 "Average Incomes of Families and Unattached Individuals, Canada, 1951-1995," Canadian Council on Social Development, www.ccsd.ca/factsheets/fs_avgin.html.
3 "A Look At Canada's Housing Performance Over Time," Huffington Post, www.huffingtonpost.ca/ypnexthome/canadas-housing-performance_b_9266608.html.
4 Population statistics drawn from Statistics Canada census data.
5 Credit Card Statistics (as of October 2015), Canadian Bankers Association, www.cba.ca/credit-card-statistics.

Spirituality Forgotten: Finding Your Post

by Yvonne Heath

In my practice I help people recover from grief, loss, and trauma. When people/parents and families do not have some kind of spiritual post, they usually feel a lot of anxiety. This is evident especially when the family experiences a death. This anxiety ripples from the parents right into the children, who will often act out their anxiety.

Yvonne and I met at a wellness show and our books have very similar titles. We both had the idea that we needed to get to know one another. Yvonne loves her life, and it shows. Her new purpose is to empower compassionate communities and professionals to live life to the fullest, learn to grieve and support others, and have 'The Talk' about end of life long before they face it.

— Elke

Spirituality is one of the most critical, and often ignored, aspects of our journey. I first understood this when I realized that I was becoming more and more anxious. Despite a 27-year nursing career, I was not well prepared for grief personally or professionally. I started having irregular heartbeats and chest pain. I even started carrying around baby aspirin, thinking that I might be having a heart attack. (If you are, baby aspirin is the first thing you will be given in an emergency room.) I was not coping well and needed change.

If we're already dealing with anxiety, why should we be talking about grief? Grief is coming. It doesn't care if we're anxious. Grief shows no mercy.

One of the most important steps I took in empowering myself during my nursing career was to go on a spiritual journey. I needed to look within and discover my values and beliefs about life and death. "How can I create a soft landing for myself, when grief arrives?"

I needed to reach out to those who could share their wisdom and help guide me to find my own internal strength; something I could hang onto in times of sadness, grief and despair. I needed to find my post, and this was my journey.

Looking at grief and anxiety from a logical point of view was my first step. The Law of Conservation of Energy states energy cannot be created or destroyed, but only changed from one form into another or transferred from one object to another. Have you ever felt the presence of someone who has died before you? A sense that they are there with you?

I believe we can stay connected and that our energy lives on. This gives me great comfort in life and in thinking about death and after death. What do you believe? What makes sense to you? Find your truth.

Our bodies do not live forever, but our love does.

Today, with the intermingling of many cultures, the freedom of choice, and the many paths available to follow, make discovering our beliefs a daunting task. You may question what you were — or were not — taught while growing up, but you may not feel that choosing your spiritual path is a task worthy of your time, or even necessary. After all, you already have enough to do every day, without adding one more thing. The difficulty with not discovering our beliefs is that when faced with challenges, we have nothing to guide us through turbulent times.

My 102-year-old friend Minnie felt she didn't have much wisdom to offer when it came to facing life's challenges. She was so wrong. When we discussed our death-phobic society and I asked what we might be missing, she looked at me with her generous smile and gentle blue eyes and said, "We all need some sort of post, something to hang onto." And there it was: the piece I was looking for.

I am convinced that Minnie was right. We all need something *internally* to hang onto when everything else is falling apart. It has to be something within: not a person, not your status, not a pet or a thing. It has to be something that you can hang onto no matter what. The most important thing you can do to manage anxiety over life's challenges is to find your post — your religion, your spirituality, yoga, or nature, whatever it may be.

Your post: that internal something that you can hang onto — no matter what — in times of despair

I have had the privilege of speaking with a variety of extraordinary and perceptive people about their understanding of life, death and grief — their posts — and I have the honour of sharing their wisdom with you.

"Thomson here!" — a minister's point of view

'Jim' is an astute retired Presbyterian minister who answers his phone, "Thomson here!" He has a mischievous smile and a devilish glimmer in his eyes. I was humbled to be invited into his home and made privy to his teachings.

Jim has known deep grief in his personal and professional life. As he was preparing to retire and travel with his lovely wife, Evelyn, she was diagnosed with cancer for the second time. Instead of a life of leisure, they faced chemotherapy and radiation. A fall eventually led to Evelyn's hospitalization, where she died two doors down from where Jim was a patient, admitted with his own health issues. Jim knows personal loss.

As a minister, Jim has led more funerals than he can recall. During a four-month period, he helped six families to cope with tragedy: three crib deaths and three teenage suicides.

He shares: "The manner in which the families were able to deal with the event often depended on whether or not there was a religious involvement that enabled the grieving to have some kind of support that provided a different overview of what happened. Those without this kind of emotional support, often provided by a religious community, had to deal with the pain in a different way that sometimes offered no broader framework within which they could understand what had taken place."

He continues, "Death comes to families in many different situations. Coming to grips with the reality and learning to survive it emotionally can depend on many factors, not least of which is how seriously people have prepared themselves to deal with death. Aging is pushed aside. Death is pushed aside. We even refuse to talk about it. We need to recognize our mortality and not be terrorized by it. We are humans, not immortals."

When people ask Jim what happens to us after death, he replies, "I haven't the foggiest, but God never turns his back on anyone and all I know is that we are going to be okay." *This is his post.*

My Mom's post

I have learned a great deal from my mother's journey over the last several decades. I am in awe of who and what she has become, and all that she strives to be, regardless of the circumstances that present themselves. Here are some of her beliefs that create her inner post.

"I am not a religious person. I am, however, a believer that I am a divine being in a physical body, experiencing life here on earth for a period of time. I choose being love and gratitude, and experiencing life and relationships with no judgment. This is my religion, so to speak. These are the soul qualities that give me a reason to get up in the morning. The more I practice being love and gratitude, the less I suffer from feelings of anger, grief and anxiety. Also, I know I am raising the vibration on this planet one loving and grateful thought or action at a time. That knowledge is my inner post, my reason for being.

"On the subject of my physical body dying, and life as I have known it coming to an end, I choose to believe that when my soul mission here is done, my spirit will leave my body. I will then go on to my next place of learning, teaching or being. My post then will continue to be love and gratitude. These are always the answers no matter what the questions.

"I see us all as lighthouses. We all have a light of love within that can shine to help guide each other along our life journeys. We can be that light if we so choose. That metaphor has helped me to hold onto my post of Being Love. This is my legacy — what I choose to leave behind, when anyone remembers my stay here and even when they don't. I know that I will have been the change that I wanted to see in the world." *This is her post.*

> **My Mom is choosing to leave behind a legacy**
> **of love and gratitude. What will your legacy**
> **be? What do you want to be remembered for?**

Derek's fiery spirit

'Derek' is the most down-to-earth, spirited United Church minister I have ever had the pleasure of calling a friend. He performs in plays, has a radio program called 'Soul Matters' and hosts a gathering of like-minded individuals at the 'Spirit Café'. He has recently completed his first novella, Dying to Live, a must-read full of spiritual insights. As a minister he pushes the boundaries, questions everything, and encourages his congregation to do the same. He considers the Bible a book of questions, not a book of answers. His honesty and integrity are a breath of fresh air.

"Church and Sunday school have not helped us with our death phobia because they have a heaven and hell story," says Derek. "This is not what I teach. That is what the church has taught for centuries and I ask, "What kind of God would do this?" I struggle with the concept that God would punish someone He loves, that the love is not stronger than anything we can do that's wrong. The question shouldn't be, "Have I done anything bad?" The question should be, "Have I done anything good?"

On the topic of spirituality versus religion, Derek says, "I think one's religion can be a part of one's spirituality, but spirituality for me has more to do with meaning and purpose. We are spiritual beings, and that means we have purpose and that can be lived out in a Christian faith or a Muslim faith, or whatever faith. The questions are inside us and the answers are inside us. We just have to sort through that and know that the answers come in many ways... "Has my life had purpose and meaning? Do I need to be forgiven or are there people I need to forgive?" These are all spiritual questions. If you have not sought your answers and made peace with yourself and others, when you are dying you will have a crisis of spirit. And no amount of pain medication can alleviate that suffering. You will be less afraid of death if you have inner peace in your life." *This is his post.*

> **If you have not sought out your answers in life**
> **— about meaning and purpose — when you**
> **are dying, you may have a crisis of spirit.**

Lela's Buddhist wisdom

My first thought after spending time with Lela, follower of Nichiren Daishonin's Buddhist teachings, was, "I want to be just like her when I grow up!" Lela exudes calmness and joy, the kind of inner peace Derek encourages us to seek in our lives. She is bright, delightful and simply a joy to be with. Lela has been a practicing Buddhist for over 25 years and has chosen the mission of helping people along their spiritual path. She accepts everyone, regardless of race, religion or sexual orientation; a lover of all people. They love her back.

In my ignorance, I believed that all Buddhists gave up their worldly goods and fun, donned a toga, and meditated for the better part of every day. I quickly learned that many of today's Buddhists are regular people who live, work and play, and have found their path to peace in these teachings.

In Buddhist philosophy, life is eternal; it has no beginning and no end. We experience one lifetime after another. Nichiren Buddhists also believe that we stay universally connected by chanting and that it is also possible to stay connected to those who have died. Consequently, death is not something to fear.

Lela says, "If you don't have any spiritual orientation you are going to be tumbling head over heels with no context, no backdrop against which to interpret the events of your life. My feeling is that people must go on a spiritual journey, and boy, they don't want to do that. Perhaps they are afraid of what they might find. So they stay in fear. If you don't want to live this way, do your spiritual work. This is your foundation. It doesn't mean you have to be a Christian, or a Buddhist, or any other religion for that matter. Find whatever spiritual belief will bring you peace in both life and death." *This is her post.*

Diane's peaceful journey through life and death

Diane was one of the most soulful people I have ever known. I had the honour and pleasure of knowing her not only as a patient in the chemotherapy clinic but as a friend.

When my husband Geordie and I married, we had our wedding pictures taken by a lake. Diane wanted to take one photo as a gift, a beautiful gesture. So she joined in, pants rolled up high, wading in the water, laughing and enjoying our celebration. Weeks later, she arrived in the clinic for a treatment and handed me the most extraordinary photo album of our special day, filled with many beautifully captured photos. I was so touched, I had to fight tears for the rest of my shift. She took lovely photos again when we were expecting our twins. She became a special part of our most precious times.

Years before, when Diane was diagnosed with cancer, she was told she had six months to live. She chose to take responsibility for her own health and did not let dying stop her from living fully. She continued to do that for 12 more years. Diane died peacefully in 2010. I met with her husband, 'Ken' to talk about the wonder of all that she *was*.

Ken shared, "Diane's eclectic spiritual beliefs intrigued me. She took what resonated with her from many different disciplines and made them her own. Her basic inner strength came from her knowledge of who she was, why she was here and where she was going. She had a belief that you can stay connected in the inner worlds and that death is not the final step. So she had no fear of dying." *This was her post.*

He added, "She was a student of learning and never stopped pursuing new knowledge. Diane was a photographer, nurse, laboratory technician, registered herbalist, cranial sacral therapist, tai chi teacher, and more. She traveled to China and learned Qigong years after her diagnosis. She loved to learn and shared her vast knowledge to help others."

Diane was a great lover of nature and organized a canoe trip for her family in her last few months of life. She also sorted her jewellery and trinkets to be given to friends and family so Ken did not have to figure it out. She also told him that she did not want him to be alone. "She made it as easy as possible for me, and for that I will always be grateful," Ken said. "She was my best friend and we stay connected in the inner worlds." *This is his post.*

The celebration of Diane's life brought joy and tears. It was held in a hall decorated with memories and her canoe. Is it surprising that Diane made all of the arrangements and enlisted many of her friends to help Ken carry out her wishes? What a selfless gift. Those who loved her shared touching stories of how inspiring she was in her life and at the end of her life. She lives on in many hearts.

Ken's final thought: "We must take responsibility, not only for our physical health, but for our spiritual health as well."

When Diane died, Ken turned to his canvas and paint to journey through his grief. In his painting, the rough water hitting the rocks depicts the turbulent times in life, and the smoother water represents the calmer days, and finally peace at the end of life.

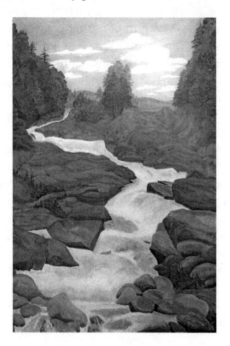

My spiritual journey, my beliefs, my post

I was raised in a Catholic home and went to church until the age of 18. When I went away to school and ventured out on my own, my spirituality took a hiatus. I thought I was far too busy to ponder such trivial things.

In my more turbulent years I truly did not have any internal beliefs to guide me. I did not have my post and so in my darkest times I suffered excessively. It wasn't until I became pregnant with our twins at age 39 that I decided it was time to choose my spiritual path — my religion — to determine my values and what I believed about life and death. Our son Tyler was 10 at the time and in a few months two more children would be born and complete our family. Someday they would ask me what I believe or I would feel compelled to teach them something valuable. I needed to find the answers that I knew were deep within. I had never questioned whether I believed in God or not.

It was just a natural part of my upbringing and it never occurred to me to question these teachings.

Then one day, while working in the emergency department, my friend and co-worker Mark and I got into one of our discussions. I was taken aback to discover that he was an atheist, the first real-life atheist I had ever known.

"You mean you really don't believe in anything?" I asked, shocked.

"Nope."

"Nothing? Really?"

"Nope. You live then you die."

And that was that. I had never heard such a thing. I needed more. I had to dig deeper. I attended various church services, speaking to priests, ministers and their congregations. I attended Buddhist gatherings, read a variety of self-help and self-discovery books, and did yoga, journaling and meditation. I spent a great deal of time in nature and talking with like-minded individuals.

One day I asked my mom's friend, Lynda, what her religious affiliation was. Her reply triggered an 'aha' moment for me. She simply asked, "Why do I have to belong to any religion?"

And therein was the final answer I was searching for. I found my 'religion'.

I believe:

+ In living a purposeful life, in being the change and in making a difference.

+ We are all connected and that everyone's well-being is everyone's concern.

+ In laughter, goodness and simplicity.

+ In random acts of kindness and bucket filling.

+ We should always leave things better than we found them.

+ It is my responsibility to become the best version of myself that I can be.

+ We all have value and should not judge anyone.

✦ We are all here for a reason, a purpose.

✦ We have no idea how long our journey will be, but it will be what it is *meant* to be.

✦ When we die, our spirits live on and we can stay connected.

✦ There is nothing to fear.

This is my religion, my spirituality. This is what I believe. *This is my post.* What do you believe? *What is your post?*

Starting your spiritual journey

Developing rituals of self-care and reflection is the key to finding inner peace, so that we can navigate through anxiety, grief and loss, and arrive on the other side feeling empowered and hopeful.

Here are 10 possible starting points for your spiritual journey.

✦ Find a peaceful place and sit quietly, even for 10 minutes a day. Just be.

✦ List your strengths, your gifts.

✦ What gives you a sense of purpose?

✦ When are you most happy, in your bliss?

✦ Seek out a mentor who has the kind of inner peace you wish for.

✦ Search for that book, course, church, gathering or counsellor. What resonates?

✦ What do you value most in your life?

✦ What are you missing in your life, and what can you do to find it or let it go?

✦ What do you need to love yourself more, to forgive yourself or others?

✦ What can you do to love life more, knowing that if you do, it will love you back?

How your spirituality can ease anxiety

A spiritual path, post or belief helps you to live a healthier life with a more positive and hopeful outlook. Here are just a few examples.

✦ Spirituality gives you something to hold onto in those times when you may feel like you have nothing else.

✦ Spirituality can relax a need to be in control or to take responsibility for everything around you.

✦ Spirituality helps you define your beliefs about life and death, and to create a soft landing for yourself when grief arrives.

✦ Spirituality connects you to something much larger than yourself, so you know in your heart that you are never alone. (Read more about this in *The Power of Connection*, page 121.)

✦ Spirituality provides an opportunity to surround yourself with like-minded others who can support you.

✦ Spirituality can give you greater resolve to deal with challenges when they arise, and a greater appreciation for good things when they happen.

✦ When you define your spirituality and how it has guided you, you have a valuable gift to share with others that could help them in their time of need. It may connect you to a greater purpose.

Brain Fitness:
For a Fit Brain and a Fit Life

by Jill Hewlett

Jill and I first connected years ago; recently I had the great pleasure of hearing her speak in person. With her passion and knowledge, I knew right away that I had to ask her to be a contributor to this book. Along with her diverse training and expertise, Jill has been licensed in Educational Kinesiology and Brain Gym® for almost two decades. I have some familiarity with these tools and have found them to be simple, accessible, and they work, which makes them favourites in my life and practice.

— Elke

Just because our morning alarm went off, our eyes are open and we're now standing upright doesn't mean our brain is fully turned on and ready for the day ahead.

Just because a deadline is approaching, a project needs completing or a decision needs to be made doesn't mean we're in a mentally clear and focused place to do it.

Just because we have people in our life we love doesn't mean we're in a place to relate, connect and enjoy each other's company.

Just because we have a head on our shoulders doesn't mean our brain is functioning and performing at its best.

It is in our power and choice to make it happen.

Anxiety can prevent us from accessing our executive functioning skills, which are required for decision-making and problem solving. We lose mental clarity and have trouble finding solutions to external issues that may be feeding the anxiety. Conversely, scientists have shown that the brain can grow, change and rewire itself to think more clearly, problem solve, uncover new perspectives, forge new initiatives, and lead new strategies.

We tend to our family, our gardens and our pets — maybe it's time for us to tend to the most powerful, sophisticated and advanced technologies on the planet, our brains?

As a highly sensitive child I was prone to anxiety and worry. This affected my confidence, body weight and quality of sleep. Gradually I learned to not only overcome, but to be empowered by these issues.

As a young adult, I made a commitment to live a life that embraces learning, growth, balance, and becoming the best I can be. It has created in me a passion for, and commitment to, helping others make positive and authentic life changes and improvements.

When I embarked on post-graduate education, I initially had plans to go into a teaching career because of my love for learning and sharing ideas. While at university I found myself filling my extracurricular time (outside of regular classes and studies) with health and wellness interests and activities.

After graduating I decided to take some time to explore other career options, ones that would encompass health and wellness goals. During this time, I began to realize that we can only teach and share these types of tools if we are willing to practice and use them in our own lives. This breeds real understanding and integrity in our work. Thus began a period of dedicated focus that I called 'My Journey'. While my journey continues today, this was a period of time during which I immersed myself like a sponge in self-development learning and holistic practices, applying them to my own needs, healing and goals.

I came to realize that while there are many pathways and approaches to health and wellness, what is essential is that we find the one(s) that resonate with us personally.

There are several therapeutic approaches that have caught my attention and in which I have spent time learning and training. However, there are two that are particularly near and dear to my heart and which have become the cornerstone components of my Brain Fitness programs: Essential Nutrients and Integrative Movement. They are the backbone of our physical, mental, emotional and functional health.

What is Brain Fitness?

The Brain Fitness program I've created is about engaging in the kinds of activities and incorporating the types of tools useful to creating a fit brain and a fit life. This training is relevant to people of all ages, and my clients range from corporate workplaces to public and private schools, boards of education, wellness centres and long-term care facilities.

The human brain is the most powerful computer on the planet. Scientists have proven that the brain can develop to a fuller capacity physically, mentally, emotionally, and functionally, so that we thrive in situations where we once struggled and become the best we can be. In fact, we are wired for this kind of meaningful growth.

Here are some typical questions I ask my audiences in my keynote and training sessions: "Are you maximizing your brain potential so you can thrive in today's world? What tools do you have to sculpt your brain and tap into your super powers?"

When we engage in the positive and effective habits that develop a fit brain, then we inevitably create a fit life.

How can improving our brain fitness helps us?

Neuroscientists have been making incredible breakthroughs and discoveries. This information has the capacity to greatly impact the growth and functioning of your brain and your life, if you have the information and know what to do with it.

Your brain can learn, develop new skills and abilities, alter behaviour and improve performance at every age with user-friendly brain fitness and wellness tools. When you change your brain, you change your results.

Here are just a few facets of our lives that we can improve through better brain fitness:

✦ *Mental health, wellness and self-care.* We can't always control what happens to us or around us, but we can control what happens within us. With mental health issues at an all time high, one of our greatest allies in effectively managing these concerns is a fit brain. The sample Brain Gym techniques described at the end of this chapter will show you how you can impact how you think, act and feel, now and in your future.

✦ *Stress resilience and change management.* Daily life stressors are not going to vanish any time soon. However, we can learn to outsmart common workplace and daily life challenges and issues by creating a fit brain. Shift yourself from reactivity to responsiveness, stress to balance and confusion to clarity.

+ *Creativity, innovation and collaboration.* The ability to change, innovate and create with ease and agility has become a critical 'must have' skill as we negotiate our lives. Brain fitness activates and grows our whole brain potential to get the results we want at work, in our relationships and in everyday life.

+ *Focus, comprehension and memory.* We can rewire and grow our brains strategically for greater results in the classroom, boardroom and daily life. Enhance project and time management, avoid procrastination, set and achieve goals, and perform at your ultimate best. Results are immediate, progressive and measurable.

How do we cultivate a fit brain?

The following two prerequisites are something our mothers have known all along but expressed in terms children understand: eat your vegetables, and go outside to play. My terminology is only a little different: get your essential nutrients, and activate your brain through movement.

1. Essential nutrition

Whatever we do to our bodies, we do to our brains. Food intake is no exception. Most people think about food to feed their bodies, but without realizing it, these very same substances are the fodder for our mental and brain health. We better make good choices!

Do you have health concerns? Have you been told that you may be predisposed to health issues due to genetics? Would you like to leverage nutrition so it has a positive impact on your physical health and mental wellbeing?

If so, then it's time to zero in on the non-negotiable brain-body fuels you require to function at your best. If you want to experience positive improvements in all areas of your life, then essential nutrition is the backbone of your success.

This has been a personal passion on my wellness journey. I have always been fascinated and affected by how food choices and consumption can make or break us — currently and in the long term.

I've spent years studying many different approaches and had the great opportunity to interview a plethora of nutrition experts on my wellness TV show. One guest in particular stood out because his knowledge and research are unparalleled.

Dr. Joel Wallach (veterinarian, pathologist, primary care physician and naturopath), was invited back as my most frequently recurring guest, as viewers learned so much from his grassroots message that for decades has been healing and reversing the health issues of people across the planet.

After the very first interview, my mother, who had been struggling with early warning signs of premature aging and disease, which were affecting her physical and mental health, decided to follow his approach. Within a few short weeks everything began to reverse and the progress continued. Almost two decades later she feels and looks better now than she did then. We hear and see these stories all the time.

Putting it to the test in my own life and with my friends, family and clients, I've learned that the 'right' essential nutrition can benefit your brain-body by:

+ Keeping your memory intact.

+ Increasing your energy levels.

+ Repairing existing health issues.

+ Improving your focus and concentration.

+ Having a more healthy and positive attitude.

+ Protecting yourself from disease.

+ Losing weight without dieting.

+ Reversing and slowing down the aging process and so much more.

Everybody needs 90 essential nutrients on a daily basis: 60 minerals, 16 vitamins, 12 amino acids and 2 essential fatty acids. These are the backbone of our health, the materials we are made of, and we must ingest them every day if we want to prevent disease, heal current issues and achieve healthy longevity.

Deriving all these nutrients on a daily basis from food alone is next to impossible. Supplementing our diets is key. After many years of research I have discovered a simple and powerful way to get these essential nutrients, and I'd be happy to share that information with those who contact me. *(See page 169 for my web address.)*

When these essential nutrients are ingested on a daily basis, seemingly miraculous changes occur, inside and out. Most of all, you will have the health, energy, stamina and vitality to live your best life and achieve your goals.

2. Integrative movement.

Nothing can optimize the body-mind connection more than movement can, because it activates the largest amount of your brain at one time. Every movement we make, from walking and talking to blinking and writing, requires intricate communication between the brain and our muscles.

When actions originate from a secure and integrated body-mind connection, an individual's natural learning abilities, confidence and sense of wellness are renewed.

Integrative movements are activities that are designed to strategically stimulate and integrate various parts of the brain, release blocks and stimulate the flow and connection between the brain centres and sensory systems, freeing the innate ability to learn and function at top efficiency.

When your body and mind work as one, you are able to perform with less stress and express yourself more effectively, using greater mental and physical potential.

Movement is also referred to as a miracle grow for the brain. According to scientific research, it also elicits higher levels of brain-derived neurotrophic factor (BDNF). This important protein influences brain function, connection and communication, as well as a variety of functions, including preserving the life span of brain cells, inducing the growth of new neurons and synapses, and supporting overall cognitive function.

By engaging in movement strategically, you can use the science of neuroplasticity to your advantage. Neuroplasticity refers to the changeability and malleability of your brain.

By using specific Brain Fitness activities, you can create new neural connections, as well as remove physical, emotional, and mental stress, invoke a more positive attitude, and develop skills and attributes such as confidence, communication, focus, problem solving, planning, decision making, and being more creative.

Whether in the classroom, boardroom or daily life, integrative movements can be used successfully to access and develop our natural abilities and achieve greater levels of efficiency, productivity and success.

> **Shift from stress to balance and re-activate**
> **and strengthen those very parts of your**
> **brain that have become disconnected,**
> **so you reconnect with your whole brain**
> **potential, and function at your best.**

Brain Gym

This is my favourite integrative movement system, and it has been the cornerstone of my personal and professional path since I first heard about it.

While it's based on modern-day neuroscience and developmental research, it's simple and easy to use, as it echoes our own natural intelligence if we were to live in better harmony with our body, nature and self-care. It can be easily and successfully used with people of all ages and stages of life, anywhere, anytime.

My mentor and dear friend Dr. Paul Dennison and his wife Gail are the co-founders of Brain Gym, a highly effective, easy to use and accessible system for people of all ages and skill levels that supports learning and development, stress resilience and goal achievement.

Dr. Dennison discovered, and proved that, "When the physical skills of learning have been mastered, the mental part can take care of itself."

Since 1981, when Dr. Dennison taught his first workshop, his work has continued to expand and grow worldwide.

Immediately after my first session, I was hooked. I couldn't believe an approach existed that spoke to our physical, emotional and mental intelligence in such clear and effective terms. The program put into words and activities an awareness that I innately knew and understood, but up to that point had never heard of or been taught. After a few years of study and practice, I became licensed in the field of Educational Kinesiology and a Brain Gym consultant. That was almost two decades ago now.

Brain Gym activities move us from using a limited portion of our brains to our whole-brain potential. They're quick, fun, and keep us energized and engaged. They can be done anywhere, any time, and are essential to our overall health and wellness.

Some common responses from my course participants are how grounded, energized, connected, and clear they feel. Everyone is excited about the abundance of tools they have learned to support their growth, self-care, stress management, emotional balance, mental clarity, communication, organization, focus, problem solving, attitude, overall well-being, and goal achievement, and to have as an additional tool in their professional toolboxes.

Experience Brain Gym

These activities to sculpt your brain are powerful and only take a few moments of your time throughout your day. Here's a three-step process to use when you are feeling stress and anxiety:

1. Rather than ignoring your body, notice how it feels and be present to any physical sensations that arise. Give your stress and anxiety levels a rating out of 1 to10 (10 being high). The act of noticing gives your mind alternative ways of thinking about and addressing a situation. When we pause and notice, we move from our habitual way of responding to creating new possibilities and new neurological connections.

2. Sip water. Your body and brain are primarily composed of water. All of the chemical actions of the brain and central nervous system are dependent on the conductivity of electrical currents between the brain and sensory organs, facilitated by water. Sipping water ensures that efficient electrical and chemical actions between the brain and the nervous system can take place.

3. Do some Brain Gym. Brain Gym activities are quick, easy and effective, and can be used anywhere, any time.

'Deepening Attitudes' is a category of specific Brain Gym activities designed to reduce stress and improve emotional balance and core postural awareness for release of the flight or fight response.

Deepening Attitudes relax the system and prepare learners to take in and process information without emotional stress.

Here are two that you can experience.

Hook-Ups

This activity, which brings both sides of the body and brain together into connection and balance, invites an experience of calm, while focusing and organizing scattered attention. As tense muscles relax, mental chatter dissipates and breathing deepens.

Notice: are you focused, organized, and able to concentrate on the task at hand, or are you easily distracted and unable to think?

Part 1: Cross your ankles. Next, extend your arms in front of you

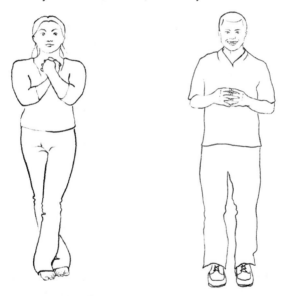

and cross one wrist (on the same side as your top ankle) over the other. Then, interlace your fingers and draw your clasped hands up towards your chest. Hold this for a minute or more, breathing slowly, with your eyes closed and the tip of your tongue on the roof of your mouth when you inhale.

Part 2: When ready, uncross your arms and legs. Put your feet flat on the floor and put your fingertips together in front of your chest, continuing to breathe deeply for another minute while holding the tip of your tongue on the roof of your mouth when you inhale.

Notice again your level of focus, organization and concentration.

What this looks like in daily life

Hook-Ups instill an overall relaxation, peace, and comfort. The person unplugs from outer world stimuli and distractions, plugging into their own inner awareness and connection. The body positioning creates a closed and connected circuitry, with an emphasis on the midline, where the physical, mental, and emotional realms can communicate and integrate.

This activity improves:

+ grounding

+ test taking

+ organization

+ assertiveness

+ accountability

+ positive energy

+ setting priorities

+ clearer listening

+ handling feedback

+ emotional centering

+ handling rejection better

+ setting and meeting goals

+ calmness and self control

+ maintaining a sense of humour

+ enhanced balance and coordination

+ data entry with speed, accuracy, and comfort

+ comfort in the immediate environment

+ managing constructive feedback

+ sense of self and boundaries

+ leaving voice mail messages

+ maintaining enthusiasm

The late Wayne Cook, a pioneering researcher of bioenergetic force fields, developed Cook's Hook-Ups, the posture from which the Brain Gym Hook-Ups were adapted, as a way to counterbalance the negative effects of electromagnetic fields. It also has the added benefit of relaxing the hip flexor muscles, while our version also emphasizes balance.

Positive points

Holding these emotional-stress release points, known as neurovascular balance points for the stomach, will invoke relaxation and calm and clear stomach aches, anxiousness and nervous butterflies.

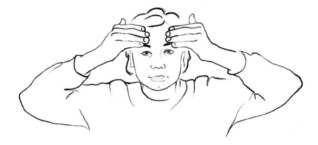

Notice whether you feel calm when performing under pressure or do you worry and get easily stressed (e.g., meeting a deadline or taking a test).

As shown in the picture, with your fingers lightly hold the two points on your forehead halfway between the hairline and the eyebrows, just above the centres of your eyes. Use just enough pressure to pull the skin taut.

Notice again your level of calm or anxiety as you think of areas of your life that may have produced stress in the past.

What it looks like in day-to-day life

The positive points access the frontal lobe to balance stress around specific memories, situations, people, places, and skills (ever forgot where you were driving to or whom you were going to call?). These points relax the reflex to act without thinking when under stress.

This activity improves:

+ reading aloud

+ positive energy

+ problem solving

+ decision making

+ public speaking

+ organizational skills

✦ sports performance

✦ staying on schedule

✦ new perspectives

✦ release of memory
  blocks

✦ test and stage
  performance

✦ handling criticism/
  rejection

✦ leadership potential

These points are the neurovascular balance points for the stomach meridian. People tend to hold stress in the abdomen, resulting in stomach aches and nervous stomachs, a pattern often established in early childhood. The Positive Points bring blood flow from the hypothalamus to the frontal lobes, where rational thought occurs. This prevents the fight-or-flight-or-freeze response, so that a new response to the situation can be learned.

Notice how you feel now. What has changed? You can anchor all the positive changes simply by noticing them.

Make sure you celebrate any changes you notice, big or small. You are on your way to creating new neurons and neural pathways.

When actions originate from the Fit Brain connection, the individual's natural learning abilities are revitalized, a relaxed and positive attitude is available, and performance becomes effortless.

Note

Brain Gym is a registered trademark of the Educational Kinesiology Foundation (Brain Gym® International) in Ventura, California. Through instructors and movement-based programs, Brain Gym® International empowers all ages to reclaim the joy of living. The organization was founded in 1987 under the name of the Educational Kinesiology Foundation and in 2000 began doing business as Brain Gym® International. Brain Gym movements, exercises, or activities refer to the original 26 Brain Gym movements developed by educator and reading specialist Paul E. Dennison and his wife and colleague, Gail E. Dennison; wzg.

Igniting Your Inner Peace Keeper

by Bari McFarland

Focusing helps elevate anxiety. In my practice and life I find when people are clear on their purpose and goals they are happier. As humans we need to feel that we are contributing and that what we do is of value. Bari's enthusiasm for helping people find their passion is exhilarating.

— Elke

"I am safe. I am safe. I am safe." Cars are whipping by me on the slushy highway. I can't believe they are going so fast when the weather is this bad. It's dark, wet and cold and I can feel my anxiety level rise as I know at any moment someone can come sliding into me or do a 360 in front of me and I'll have to hit my brakes.

"I am safe. I am safe. I am safe." This is my mantra during my long commute to work.

Hi. My name is Bari McFarland and I'm a commuter. I don't like big cities and the hustle and bustle of all the people, so I choose to live in a smaller city over an hour away from my job. Here I am in my car every morning at 6:00 a.m., making my way in to the city with thousands of other people. People who don't know how to drive.

This was my life for years. Getting up at 5:00 a.m. so that I could go to the gym before work, making the 1.5- to 3-hour drive to a job that was sucking the life out of me (more about that later), and then making my long way back home only to arrive famished, stressed and angry. I'd walk in the door, to shoes, clothes and a school bag littering the front hall. I'd immediately call out to my son Cody to come pick up his things.

It wasn't until my husband Ken pointed it out to me that I became aware that my first interaction with him and Cody each day was full of anger, frustration and negative energy. They were asleep when I left for work, and when I got home the first thing I did was to lash out.

When Elke invited me to contribute a chapter to this book, I immediately said yes. I had experienced different levels and forms of anxiety every day. Not only in commuting to and from work, but sitting in meetings hoping people wouldn't find out I really didn't know what I was doing. However, I had three things going for me: I wanted to do something about my anxiety, I knew I had the power to do it, and eventually I found a solution that has ignited my inner peace keeper and reinvigorated my life. Now I want to help you do the same.

Since my late teens I've been interested in personal development and wanted to know why I did the things I did and thought what I thought. I learned early on that I was powerful and the only person responsible for creating my reality. If there was something in my life I didn't like or want, it was my responsibility to change it. Knowing this didn't mean everything was easy. On the contrary, I was constantly in my head, always analyzing what I thought and felt.

When Ken brought to my attention that I was a crazy person when I got home from work, I wanted to know why. I started to notice what I was thinking on my drive home. I listened to the voice inside my head when I walked in the door and saw the mess. I was mad. I was jealous. Here I was with a great husband, amazing kid, good job, and yet I wasn't happy. I had to commute and work long hours and my husband got to stay home, do work he loves on his schedule, take naps, and be there for Cody when he came home from school. I wanted some of that and I needed help to get it.

So off to the self-help section of the bookstore I went, where I came across an amazing book called *The Passion Test — The Effortless Path to Discovering Your Life Purpose*, by Janet Bray Attwood and Chris Attwood. I loved it so much I became a Passion Test facilitator. Teaching others and going through the processes myself helped me learn at a deeper level the principles of the law of attraction and how important it is to get clear about what you want.

The law of attraction tells us that what we think about affects how we feel, and how we feel emits an energy/vibration that goes out into the world and attracts back that which is like itself. Everything outside of ourselves is first created within. So, if I wasn't happy I first needed to ask myself what would make me happy and then create it.

This is where *The Passion Test* comes in and the formula I live and breathe on a daily basis. Embodying these three simple words has helped to reduce my anxiety and manifest a life I couldn't have imagined five short years ago:

INTENTION
ATTENTION
NO TENSION

Intention

This is the 'what'. What do you want? What does it look like, feel like, taste like when you are living your life full out? The first step in creating the kind of life you want is to get really clear on the 'what'. If you don't know what you want, how are you going to manifest it?

I remember one of the first times I put this principle into practice during my commute. I was going over a conversation I'd had with a colleague at work. I hadn't seen her in a couple of years and one day, passed her in the hall. She asked me how I was doing and if I was enjoying my new job. I remember saying, "I'm great, I love my job!" I got back to my office and thought, "What? No I didn't." In fact, I hated it. I was in a management position responsible for an area I had no experience or training in, basically learning as I went along. I had people reporting to me who, I felt, knew a heck of a lot more than I did.

So, I woke up each day and put a mask on. The mask covered up the fact I that didn't have a university degree and someone was going to find out. The mask portrayed a happy, I-can-do-anything kind of attitude. The mask covered up the real me and the real life I wanted. I didn't know what this was because I didn't let myself think about it. The only thing the mask didn't cover was the anxiety welling up inside me.

After going over how much I wasn't enjoying my job, I added, "I hate commuting. I hate getting up at 5:00 a.m. and not getting home till 7:00 p.m." I thought, Okay, if this isn't what I want, then what do I want? My answer: "I want to work close to home, I want to eat meals with my family, I want to do work I love, I want to live on the water."

Now picture a car going 100 miles an hour and listen as it comes to a screeching halt. This was the sound I heard in my head when I tried to figure out how it was going to happen. Limiting beliefs showed up, such as "There aren't any good jobs in my city, I can't quit, we need the benefits, and we can't afford a house on the water." No wonder I didn't ask myself what I wanted. In my mind there was no way I could have it.

Then I remembered something I read in *The Passion Test*. Worrying about how it's going to happen gets in the way of what we want.

So we need to put the 'how' aside and get clear on the 'what'. Don't worry, the 'how' is important. Believe me. As much as I believe in the law of attraction, I also believe we need to take action and not sit around twiddling our thumbs. The 'how' comes later and I'll talk about that, but first, let's get clear on the 'what'.

I highly recommend picking up *The Passion Test* and taking yourself through the exercises Janet and Chris share. In the meantime, I've created an exercise to help you get started on getting clear right now and igniting that inner peace maker.

Exercise: Creating a dream book

I'm not talking about the ones that happen when you sleep. I'm talking about the ones you create when you're awake. For now, just grab a blank sheet of paper. However, if you have a journal you can reserve for this purpose, use that.* Next, pick a pen that fits comfortably in your hand and glides over the page. There is something about handwriting that connects the brain to what you've written. It helps to clarify your thoughts, makes them stick, and makes it easy to pull out later when you can't remember what it was that you wanted.

I started my dream book with "Dreams come true for me and you." The 'you' part refers to my inner child or spirit/soul within. You may want to start with your favourite quote or something else that inspires and makes you feel good. If you can't think of anything right now, leave a blank space and fill it in later.

On the next line write the sentence "I am...". The "I am" statement brings us into the energy of here and now, and because our brains don't know fact from fiction, the message our bodies receive is that what we want is already happening. It makes us feel good. If we say, "I want" or "I wish", it has a tendency to make us feel that what we want is out there, out of reach. Our brains then think of all the reasons why it's not going to happen and this creates a lower vibration. Make sense? Let's get started.

Pretend you have a magic wand and you can do, be, and have anything you want. Think of all the different areas of your life: your career, relationships, hobbies, how you'd like to feel, your health, etc. Finish the statement, 'I am'. Here are some of my examples. I am:

---

* The Artist's Reply has a beautiful one you can purchase. Please refer to the end of the book.

✦ In a loving, intimate relationship with my husband.

✦ Enjoying a close relationship with my son.

✦ Living in a beautiful home on the water.

✦ Feeling confident, happy and enjoying life.

✦ Trusting that where I am is where I'm supposed to be.

✦ Helping others live more joyful lives.

The most important part is to feel good. You want what you've written to create a high vibration. If it doesn't make you feel good, change the statement. For example, if you are in an abusive relationship and you've written "I am in a loving, respectful relationship" but right now you just can't see how that's possible, don't write it. At this point, "I am dating," "I feel loved," or "I am having a quiet day to myself" may be what makes you feel good. Doing this not only creates a higher level vibration, it puts you into the frame of mind for taking action. Which brings us to the second part of the formula, attention.

Attention

What are you putting your attention on? The Passion Test talks about two aspects of attention, but I like to add a third one. They are:

a. what are you thinking about

b. what actions are you taking

c. whose business are you in?

This is where "how is it going to happen" comes in, the "I know what I want, now what?"

Let's start with a) what are you thinking about?

If you would like to be in a loving relationship, but all you think about is that there aren't any good men/women out there, dating is hard, you have no time, etc., then that's what you'll keep getting and you won't take the action necessary to meet someone. Make sense?

So, notice where you are putting your attention. When I thought about wanting to live on the water and work close to home and heard myself say, "You can't afford that" or "There aren't any good jobs up here," I reminded myself of this part of the formula. I knew my job was to get clear and focus on what I wanted, rather than what I didn't want.

That's when things started to open up, allowing me to b) take action. For instance, I was having my regular Sunday morning chat with my mom and she mentioned a cottage my step dad had for sale on a lake just north of us and asked if we'd like to see it. I could have just said no. Remember, I can't afford to live on the water. But something in me said, "Okay, let's just be open to this." Well, to make a long story short, we saw it and bought it.

And that's not the end of the story. A few short months later, I was having a conversation with my boss about the stress I was feeling due to commuting and that I was applying for jobs closer to home. He suggested I work from home a couple of days a week. What? I hadn't even considered that that could be an option.

Which brings me to c) staying in my own business. Byron Katie, another mentor of mine, talks about three kinds of business:

✦ your business — what you think, say and do

✦ my business — what I think, say and do

✦ God's business — all the things you can't control, like the weather

When I wondered what other people would think, I was in other people's business. Well, Bryon Katie says when you're in someone else's business, there's no one in yours. So I got back into mine and told myself I'd probably get more work done at home than I did at work, without all the interruptions. And that's exactly what happened.

Before I knew it, I was waking up without an alarm four days a week, living on the water, and commuting to the city three days. I never would have believed it. Actually, this is where I need to say I did believe, in my heart and soul, that what I wanted on that list would happen, I just didn't know how or when. I just knew I needed to get clear about what I wanted, focus on it, and let go. Yes, let go, the no-tension part of the formula.

No tension

This part is sometimes the hardest. Letting go. Acting from that place of peace and calm, the place of knowing, that what you want (all those things you listed in your dream book) will show up, you just may not know how or when. No tension is about being open to what shows up in your life, and using those times when things don't work out to get clear about what you want.

I think back to when I first became a Passion Test facilitator. I was working full time and still commuting three days a week. I had decided to start my coaching business and planned to do it part time until I retired. I remember being so stressed out with everything on my plate. Each night I'd come to bed and ask myself, "What the heck am I thinking?" I'd have this conversation in my head:

"What is your intention?"

"To help people discover their passion."

"Do you believe that will happen?"

"Yes."

"What are you putting your attention on? Are you focusing on what you want and are you taking action?"

"Yes. I am thinking positively and about what I want, visualizing and feeling it in my body as if I already have it, and I am taking action. I'm doing everything I can think of to move my business forward and manage my full time job."

"Okay Bari, then let go (the 'no tension' part). Be open to how and what is showing up."

By the time I told myself to let go, I could feel the stress leaving my body. I would go to sleep and when I woke up something wonderful would have happened. Has this ever happened to you? When you allow yourself to let go, somehow, some way, it works out.

It's crazy to think about my life now compared to a short five years ago. Everything on my list has shown up. I wake up without an alarm, on a beautiful 45-acre property on the water. I work from home doing what I love — helping others connect more deeply with their true selves and live more joyful lives. I am more in love with my husband today than ever because I love me more. My son and I are more connected today because I am more connected with myself. When my anxiety shows up (which it does), I embrace it rather than resist it and use it for me rather than against me.

As I wrap up this chapter, I invite you, when feeling anxious, to start noticing your thoughts. Use it as a signal to stop, go within, and embrace what you are feeling. Ask yourself, are you thinking more about what might happen, rather than what you want to have happen? Use the formula of 'intention, attention, no tension' to bring yourself back on track. Keep your dream book handy, read it every day, and feel it in your body as if it's already happened. When something happens that you don't want, flip it around to what you do want and add it to your list. Remember, everything outside ourselves is first created within.

From my heart to yours. May you love and embrace all of you, and live your life authentically, fully and on purpose.

The Power of Connection

by Suzanne Witt-Foley

Suzanne describes connection so well. When we feel separate we suffer. Whether we practice The Course in Miracles, Buddhism, or any kind of spirituality, we are 'pack animals' and meant to be in groups/community/tribes. We need to know that we belong somewhere.

— Elke

Dominican Republic — Mission Trip 2010

As we bumped our way along a dusty dirt path, sun blazing down on us, I thought about how to prepare for the experience that I would have along with 20 other mission volunteers, as this first day in the Dominican Republic began to unfold. We sat in the back of an open air bus, packed tight like sardines alongside hockey bags filled with shoes, medicine and hygiene products.

We were making our way to remote and isolated Haitian refugee villages. Haitian refugees living in the Dominican Republic are among the most poverty stricken, oppressed people in the world. Homes are essentially dirt floor shacks with scrap metal forming the walls and rooftops. People live hand to mouth, often not knowing where their next meal will come from or when. Haitian refugees are not allowed to work and children may not attend school unless their parents can pay for it, which few can. The people of these villages have come to rely on voluntary groups such as Dominican Crossroads, the mission group that I travelled with, to provide basic necessities for survival: food, clothing and basic medical care.

As we were jostled about, en route to our first stop, I thought about the impact that such difficult circumstances can have on people. Given my long-time career in the field of mental health and addictions, I was keenly aware that poverty and mental illness can often go hand in hand, and substance use can sometimes provide the only escape or temporary relief from the relentless struggle for survival. I expected to see hopelessness, desperation and despair. I expected to see people ravaged by illness and addictions.

I could not have been more surprised. As we pulled into the first community and the bus came to a stop, children came running. They skipped down the road wearing ear-to-ear grins and a palpable sense of joy. As we unloaded from the bus they gathered round, reached out to hold our hands and, although they did not speak English, called us 'friend'.

As the week unfolded and we visited village after village, it became obvious to me that my model for mental health did not fit these circumstances. Instead of helplessness, here was a strong sense of community, connection and hope all woven into the fabric of daily life. Everyone cared for one another. Parents, grandparents, teens and other children cared for the littlest ones and one another. No one was left behind. Every 'door' was open.

A Piece of Candy

One day, after we had given out all of our 'wares', I searched around for just one more thing to give to the little girl who had been walking with us. In the depths of my pack I found one little wrapped candy. As I handed her the candy, her face lit up. She unwrapped it, placed it in her teeth, and cracked it into her hand. The candy had broken apart into many little pieces. She then turned to her friends and gave each and every one of them a tiny shard of candy.

Over and over again, I bore witness to incredible acts of kindness, sharing, caring and love. Over and over again, I was stuck by the stark contrast between what I expected to see and what I experienced.

One day I was talking with our guide about the work I do back home. I spoke about the prevalence of mental illness and increasing concerns about escalating mental health issues and addictions. He seemed surprised. "We don't really see very much mental illness here in these villages. I see very few people struggling with depression or anxiety. And in fact, we see virtually no issues with addiction."

Why were these disadvantaged people, thrust into the backwaters of human civilization due to political strife and impoverishment, not experiencing the great stress on human psyches that seemed so imminent? That mission trip for me was the beginning of a journey toward a new understanding of mental health, the powerful protective effect of connection, inclusion and relationships, and how a broader sense of hope, belonging and community contribute to well-being.

When I speak at conferences or workshops, I will often start by asking the audience to reflect on the world we live in. I ask people how the way we live today has changed compared to when they were children.

People comment on the many ways our 'culture' has changed. More women have joined the workforce, creating a need for child daycare. People work longer hours. Divorce and single-parent families are more prevalent. Families are smaller, homes are typically bigger.

People also comment on how childhood has changed. Outside of school hours, young people are less likely to be out exploring their physical worlds with others and more frequently found at home, alone, sitting in front of a screen. In fact, technology has made a significant impact in how all of our daily lives unfold. One hundred years ago, only eight percent of homes had a telephone. Today 80 percent of homes have Internet access. Even in the last five to ten years, technology has changed the way we relate, communicate and connect with one another.

We are more socially disconnected and isolated, and have less human-to-human contact. We have more electronic connection and less human touch connection.

We are seeing an unprecedented speed of change in the history of humanity. We have seen more rapid change in the last century than any other century in the history of human existence.

I propose that we have likely seen more change in this past decade than any other decade of human existence.

One difficulty is the speed of this change relative to our human evolution. Many of us might believe that we can adapt and be flexible to the rapidly changing culture in which we live. However, evolution is the very reason we are not able to adapt and thrive.

We cannot possibly adapt in the short term because evolution requires generations of time for living organisms to streamline and adapt to a particular environment. We lived as hunters and gatherers for over 200,000 years. Human beings are highly evolved for this lifestyle because for generation after generation our brains and bodies have been adapting to this environment to ensure our survival. However, we live today within a culture that has never been further removed from that lifestyle.

I propose that there are two driving forces still residing within all of us, gifted from this historic way of life: the drive for survival and the need for connection.

Human brain circuitry is finely tuned and streamlined for survival. Our 'fight or flight' fear response, or 'stress response' system, has been designed to become engaged any time we feel our survival is threatened. Imagine yourself at a cave-person campfire when suddenly a sabre-toothed tiger intrudes. Instantly the fear or stress response kicks in to aid in survival. Adrenaline and other stress hormones begin to circulate through the bloodstream. The heart begins racing; blood pressure escalates, pumping oxygen and nutrients to the muscles to strengthen them for battle or escape. Digestion slows down; the brontosaurus burger in our bellies can wait. The immune system lowers. We don't need it at the moment to fight off some dreaded disease. We need all sources of energy to 'feed, fight, or flight'.

This can explain the stories we sometimes hear of heroic strength. We read in the news: 'Man Lifts Car Off Trapped Person'. This shouldn't be humanly possible, but it may be the result of the superhuman strength that the 'fight or flight' response can provide.

This is all very good if our lifestyles involve just the odd sabre-toothed tiger attack. What science has revealed to us, however, is that the culture we live in today is chronically and toxically turning on these survival mechanisms. Under this constant bombardment, the system constantly recalibrates and the stress becomes toxic. This may well be the root of chronic disease such as diabetes, cancer and heart disease, as well as mental illnesses such as anxiety, depression, Post Traumatic Stress Disorder (PTSD) and addiction.

Most of us are able to manage and handle stress in the short term. In fact, we can manage a fair bit. But if we are holding on to our stress day and night or taking a break from our stress, eventually it will become the focus of our lives. It will cause us excruciating pain, and all other elements that bring us joy and meaning will become unimportant.

Now consider our survival response. How did we live as hunter/gatherers? Were we all alone out in the forest? Of course not. We lived in groups or tribes. Human beings stayed together for survival.

We are pathetically ill-equipped to survive all alone. We don't have sharp claws like a bear, fangs like a wolf, or the grace and speed of a deer. No quills, no fur, not even a particularly bad smell. As humans, the only reason we survived those 200,000 years is because we stayed together. Because unity provided us with safety. We cared for and protected one another to ensure our survival.

When we feel connected, included, and part of the group, our brains register that we are safe. When we feel safety, it takes us out of stress response. Human beings are social animals — our brains are wired that way to ensure survival. We feel safety and security when we feel connected, nurtured, included, when we have people to care for and people who care about us; when we feel that we belong to a clan or tribe.

We are starting to recognize this driving force and the importance of our social well-being as a contributor to our overall health. Recently, I had the opportunity to hear Matt Lieberman speak — a social neuroscientist from University of California, Los Angeles (UCLA).[1] He asks the question: "What are one or two of the most painful experiences of your life?"

Think about that. Answer the question in your own mind. Some of you might be thinking of a broken leg, a fall, or childbirth. Others might be thinking about the loss of a loved one, a relationship break-up, or perhaps some kind of public humiliation, such as declaring bankruptcy.

For some of you, a physical pain may have come to mind; for others, a social pain. Pain signals us to pay attention; it tells us there is a threat to our survival. What we now know is that social pain, just like physical pain, also triggers the stress response. We tend to believe that social and physical pain are different, yet our brains do not differentiate. Social pain and physical pain both activate the same region of the brain (dorsal anterior cingulate cortex). Both signal a threat to survival. Our social attachments function by piggybacking onto the physical pain system.

When we ask people to list their top 10 fears, the results fall into three categories: physical harm or death (threat to survival), death or loss of loved one (threat of isolation equals threat to survival), and speaking in public.

What are we afraid of when speaking in public? We are afraid of rejection because rejection hurts. Many of us experience classic 'fight-or-flight' sensations before making a speech or speaking in public: heart racing, sweating, rapid breathing, nausea, running to the bathroom several times; all are signs of anxiety. Rejection is a perceived threat to our survival. Is public speaking a real threat to our longevity? Perhaps not, but try convincing our primitive brains to listen to reason under such stress. These concepts help us to understand the power in bullying, discrimination, racism, and stigma. We all have a need to belong. Signs that we are liked, admired, loved, treated fairly, and praised, are all signs that we belong.

Let's talk about anxiety. What is anxiety? Anxiety is fear. It is future focused fear. Anxiety disorder is essentially a situation when the fight-or-flight response has been 'recalibrated' and 'dysregulated', and 'fight-or-flight' is triggered to such a degree that it begins to inter-fere with a person's ability to function day to day: to work, go to school, and maintain healthy relationships. The trick to managing anxiety is to find a set of strategies that help diminish stress response, and help the brain recognize that there is safety rather than threat.

We live in a culture where there has been an insidious rise in indi-vidualism and isolation. Throughout human history we could take the value of our connectedness for granted, because it simply was built into our way of life. Today, we need to find ways to consciously connect with one another in order to preserve our sense of safety and protect our health and well-being. How may we accomplish this?

Finding solutions

Michael Lambert, a psychology professor at Brigham Young Univer-sity, reviewed 40 years of research to identify the elements of therapy that bring a person from a place of struggle to a place of well-being[2]. What is it about therapy, he asks, that helps a person move along the path to recovery?

Lambert found that more than 70 percent of 'what works' is rela-tional in nature. Relationships, connection, and belonging promote a sense of safety and calm the brain. How can we apply this to our day-to-day lives?

The people I have met who manage their mental health most effec-tively have built a solid support system for themselves. Their support system includes family members, friends, self-help groups, therapy, and support groups. They are also connected to and involved in their communities, participating in sports, book clubs, and bridge clubs. They actively volunteer with their faith groups, service clubs, hospi-tals, or in the mental health field itself. They have found places where they feel included and a sense of belonging, and they have found opportunities to care for and support others. At the risk of sound-ing repetitive, this is how we are built. When we have opportunities to care for one another, we are able to foster a sense of safety and well-being.

Tips for deepening our connections

Although there are many effective strategies for managing anxiety, let's focus on strategies that apply connections and relationships to mitigate the stress response and enhance our sense of safety.

1. **Create a list of people in your closest circle who love you and support you.** It may include a significant other, parents, siblings or other relatives, and close friends or colleagues. Think about your past and include people who have been there for you (or you for them). Notice that you may have distanced yourself from some or many of them.

2. **Create a checklist (with time frames) of ways in which you could reconnect or strengthen these ties.** Examples could include:

   ✦ Committing to a weekly phone/Skype call to reach out to someone. Place a reminder in your cell phone or on your calendar to ensure that you follow through.

   ✦ Inviting a friend for a walk, for coffee, or to plan, prepare and share a meal together.

   ✦ Sending a card in the mail (the old-fashioned way) just to say "Hi" and let them know you are thinking of them.

   ✦ Buying, making or baking a small gift for someone and taking it to them.

   ✦ Inviting someone to go to a movie or to spend time with you watching your favourite funny sitcom episodes. Invite them to make it a weekly or monthly event with you.

Start small. Commit to making one phone call to a sibling or friend you haven't talked to in a while.

3. **Create a list of interests and activities you enjoy.** Next, brainstorm a list of ways that you can grow your involvement with other people in these activities. Explore opportunities in your community and create a checklist (with timeframes) of your goals. For example:

+ If you enjoy running, find a friend who would be interested in joining you to train for a 5k running event. Join a running club or sign up for a 'learn to run' course offered at the community centre.

+ If you enjoy reading, consider a book club (join one or create your own with just a couple of friends), or invite a friend to the library and together pick a book that you will both read and spend time discussing.

4. **Consider what you are passionate about, where you would like to make a difference in this world, or how to make a contribution to your community or neighbourhood.** Again, create a list and begin to explore opportunities, providing yourself with steps to take and timeframes. Examples could include:

+ Joining a faith group or service club.

+ Volunteering at the hospital, a seniors' home or assisting in coaching a team.

+ Becoming a Big Brother/Sister.

+ Hosting a BBQ or planning a progressive dinner or potluck meal with your neighbours.

Start small. Maybe the first thing you do is mow an elderly neighbour's lawn, bake them some cookies, or shovel their driveway.

Remember that none of these strategies is easy and they can seem overwhelming. They take time, commitment and energy. Try not to bite off more than you can chew. Success will come if you start small and slowly build your connections and relationships.

Tips for deepening the connection within ourselves

It's not only about connecting at community and relational levels. It's also about deepening the connection within ourselves. "The greatest sources of suffering are the lies we tell ourselves," says Bessell van der Kolk, a leading trauma psychiatrist.[3] Our lived experience shapes how we view the world and how we fit in it (or don't fit in it).

Throughout our lives we receive constant messaging from our parents, family members, teachers, schools, workplace and broad culture about how we should be, look, feel, or not feel. This messaging often cultivates competitiveness and emphasizes our separateness. As a result, many of us are highly self critical and have these little voices in our heads that tell us things like "I am too fat," "I have no friends," "I'm a bad mother," "I'm not smart enough," "I'm not good enough."

We create isolation or separation even within our own minds. Perhaps the first place to build connections, safety, and security is within ourselves.

1. **Cut yourself some slack.** Be kind to yourself. Give yourself the same kindness and care that you would give a good friend. This is called self compassion. Think about what you would say to a friend if they were struggling with anxiety. Say the same kind of things to yourself. For example, you might say to a friend, "Sounds like things are really hard for you right now. It's going to be okay. Things will get better. People do recover. You will too." Tell yourself these things. Writing down these compassionate statements can also help.

2. **An important element of self compassion is cultivating self awareness or mindfulness.** If we don't notice our self criticism, then we can't give ourselves the compassion we need. Notice those critical statements we say to ourselves. Replace them with more compassionate statements. Validate your own experience.

3. **Recognize our common humanity and our shared imperfect human experience.** To be human is to suffer, but to feel isolated and alone in our suffering is significantly more painful.

For me, the mission trip to the Dominican Republic was the beginning of a journey toward a better understanding of the powerful protective effect of connection, inclusion and relationships, and how a broader sense of hope, belonging, and community contribute to well-being.

Social connectedness is a powerful mitigator of toxic or unrelenting stress. It may, in fact, be the most powerful protective factor and regulator of the stress response system. For our highly paced, stress-induced society, it may just take a few impoverished villages full of healthy, caring people to lead the way.

How Connection and Relationships Can Ease Anxiety

Inclusion, belonging and relationships help to promote a sense of safety and reduce the experience of anxiety. Here's how.

+ When we feel connected, included, nurtured and loved, our brains register that we are safe.

+ Feeling safe is the opposite of feeling threatened.

+ Anxiety is our threat response or fear response turning on.

+ Fostering a sense of safety is a powerful way to mitigate the fear response and reduce anxiety.

+ Creating opportunities to surround yourself with people who care about you, people who support you and/or share common interests, tells the brain that you are safe and reduces the experience of anxiety.

Notes

1. Mathew Dylan Lieberman, PhD, is an award-winning professor and social cognitive neuroscience lab director at UCLA's Department of Psychology, Psychiatry and Biobehavioral Sciences. He conducts research into the neural bases of social cognition and social experience, with particular emphasis on the neural bases of emotion regulation, persuasion, social rejection, self-knowledge, theory of mind, and fairness.
2. Michael J. Lambert, PhD, specializes in mood measuring and behaviour change. He has authored or co-authored several books on methodology for clinical psychologists.
3. Bessel A. van der Kolk, M.D. has been the Medical Director of The Trauma Center in Boston for the past 30 years. He is a Professor of Psychiatry at Boston University Medical School and serves as the Co-Director of the National Center for Child Traumatic Stress Complex Trauma Network. He is Past President of the International Society for Traumatic Stress Studies.

Creative Practices

My personal invitation to you: awareness and practice

Over the years, personally and professionally, I have learned that we need to check in with ourselves, our body, mind, spirit, and emotions every day. Only with awareness are we able to change and learn.

I have learned that we need to be consistent in order to be successful. Practice makes our new habits comfortable. We need to take care and nurture each part, daily. When we do this, we can be balanced and happier. When we cope better, we are able to add more value when helping others. With regular self-care, we can give a more enriched experience to others.

There are many ideas here. Try, explore, and play. Discover the ones you like and the ones that give you the most energy. Make your daily practice your own. Everybody is uniquely, beautifully different, so that means different strategies work for different people.

Whatever your 'combination' is, make it your own and practice it daily. You will experience a difference and this will help make you feel better, as it has for many others before you. At the end of this chapter is a support chart that you can personalize.

The more connected you are to yourself, the more connected you are to your world.

CREATIVE PRACTICE 1:
Identifying your mental blocks

In the list below, check off those mental blocks that feel familiar and, in some cases, justified:

❏ Competition

❏ Time

❏ Money

❏ Lack of knowledge

❏ Opinion

❏ Lack of gratification

❏ Lack of support

❏ Distractions

❏ Fear

❏ Rituals

❏ Belief systems

❏ Habits

❏ Cultural beliefs

❏ Patterns

❏ Judgment

❏ Perfectionism

❏ Fear of change

❏ Fear of failure

❏ Fear of success

❏ Addiction

❏ Obsessions

❏ Resentments

❏ Work ethic

❏ Overwork

❏ Emotional blocks, walls, fears

❏ Wanting to be perfect

❏ Wanting the project to be 'right'

❏ Policies, rules, procedures, protocol

Name and describe what you believe is standing in the way of your dreams, your creativity, or loving your life. If you have personal blocks missing from the list, add them.

Consider the blocks you defend.

Make a list of ways to eradicate all or part of a block with the resources you have today. Include in that list the steps you can take in the next few days, in the next few weeks, and even months ahead.

What one small step can you take now?

If you have trouble articulating your blocks and steps, try the 'Facing the Dragon' and 'Block Busters' exercises below.

CREATIVE PRACTICE 2:
Facing the Dragon

What would you need to face the dragon? Are you holding back on something you do not want to face? Perhaps this is a clear signal to look at that challenge in depth. What can you learn here?

Ask yourself these questions and write your answers:

✦ Do you know what stresses you?

✦ Is it confrontation?

✦ Is it financial?

✦ Is it commitment?

✦ Is it the unknown results of any type of change?

✦ What is it that you don't want to experience?

✦ What experience will help to overcome it?

✦ What is it that you are afraid will happen?

✦ Is there a problem?

✦ What would help you overcome the fear?

✦ What might change in your life?

✦ What is there to gain or lose?

✦ Will you have to accept something?

✦ Will it affect your family life?

✦ Will it affect your work?

✦ Does it challenge your belief system? Is it possible that one of these answers is creating resistance to overcoming a block and pursuing a dream?

CREATIVE PRACTICE 3:
Block busters

Break through your blocks by working through the following questions. Give yourself as much time as you need, answering in point form.

+ Is a block/belief stopping you from pursuing a dream?

+ Is it manageable or unmanageable? State how in either case.

+ What would small steps look like?

+ What step can you take now toward surpassing your block to be closer to your dream?

+ What step can you take tomorrow?

+ Can you take the time to imagine how it will feel when you reach your goal?

+ Can you take the time to imagine how it will feel once you overcome your block?

+ What step can you take this week?

+ What step can you take this month?

+ How will you support yourself?

+ Who and what will support you with your steps?

+ Is there someone you can share your goals with?

Stimulating your perceptions

Take your block busting a step further with these three practices:

+ Try journaling, as described in *Creative Practices*, number 15.

✦ Try painting the essence of your block.

✦ Try painting the essence of your goal.

Describe the differences and similarities in your two paintings. How can these differences and similarities relate to any of your notes on blocks?

CREATIVE PRACTICE 4:
Questions about choice

Write down your answers to the following:

✦ What do I think about my situation?

✦ What are my choices? (Feel free to list any and all choices that come to mind, judging none, as this is a work list and you empower yourself with choices. The next questions help you to edit those choices.)

✦ Is this a choice good for me now?

✦ Does this choice come from fear? From anger? From guilt? From love?

✦ How do I feel emotionally? Physically?

✦ Is there a better choice for me?

✦ What do I need?

✦ Is this choice good for my family?

✦ Is there a choice that benefits everyone?

✦ Which options give me the most inner peace?

Visualize each choice and some possible outcomes. How does each choice feel? Any surprises?

Consider the source of each feeling in order to understand, rather than defend it. Feelings are real, they cannot be denied. Accept them; understand them.

✦ Is the feeling a fight-or-flight-or-freeze reaction?

✦ Is this a feeling from a past experience? How far past — recent or childhood?

✦ Is the feeling based on a belief system?

Now, after you have done all this, ask yourself, "Will my choice serve me well and enhance my life (and possibly the lives of those around me)?" And again, ask yourself, "Which choice will give me the most inner peace?"

CREATIVE PRACTICE 5:
Staying present: Five senses

This is a wonderful exercise that helps lower anxiety and panic. Use the scale 0 to10 to measure your anxiety level. Try this exercise and then measure again. Use your five senses. It does not matter in which order you do them.

✦ Look at three objects around you. For each object name three descriptive qualities; for example, a lamp with a beige lampshade, long brass stem and round base.

✦ Note three sounds, then note three smells — your clothes, paper, a book, it does not matter. Notice how they are different from each other.

✦ Note three textures. Linger in the differences, rough, silky, smooth, and so on.

✦ Note three tastes, or perhaps one taste with three aspects. For example, chocolate — soft creamy, definite, nutty.

✦ Now recall the three objects you first looked at.

✦ Check your level of anxiety, 0 to 10.

When I have done this exercise with a group, peoples' anxiety goes down. You can repeat this exercise until your anxiety level is manageable again. In my office, we have made up sensory bags for young people containing small objects to stimulate the five senses.

CREATIVE PRACTICE 6:
Yes/no/maybe exercise

I learned this exercise from a few workshops and facilitators. The purpose is to help you learn your body cues.

Pair up with your partner, your children, or a friend. One person remains stationary and is the receiver. The other person is the doer, and gently taps, rubs or shakes the receiver in various places, repeating each motion so the receiver can monitor the sensation and reply with "Yes" when they like it, "No" when they don't, and "Maybe" when they are not sure, in which case the doer can repeat the action a bit longer. Each person gets 10 minutes.

CREATIVE PRACTICE 7:
Tree meditation (grounding)

Grounding yourself and staying connected to your body enables you to handle more emotional states. It helps you to be more aware of your surroundings, feel stronger and rooted.

You can do this exercise with your eyes open, soft eyes (partially open eyes) or closed, standing, lying down or in a seated position. You may want to record this and then listen to it to get more benefit.

1. **Take a moment to notice your body and your breathing.** There is no need to change your breathing, just notice.

2. **Imagine yourself as a tree, your body as the trunk.** As you breathe, imagine that your legs are growing roots through the floor, and past any other materials into the earth. Each breath extends and grows your roots. These roots explore the earth and meet aquifers, other roots, animals, bugs, ants, and so on. Each breath feels connected to other roots and the earth. Slowly take your breath into your body, letting the roots soak in the nutrients of the earth, letting the earth feed you, bringing your breath into your trunk. Your breath is now coming up through your roots and into your trunk.

3. **Slowly change your breathing, inhaling from your trunk into your arms, which grow into branches.** Reaching to the sky, each breath grows leaves. Notice the warm sun on your branches and the wind through your leaves. Let

yourself experience being the tree. Then slowly change your breathing, imagine taking the air into your branches and into your trunk, feeling fed by the sun, the rain, the wind.

4. **Slowly alternate the direction of your breathing.** Inhale and feel your neck, head, and arms as the crown of the tree, moving into branches and leaves. Then exhale into your torso as the trunk of the tree and feel your legs and feet as the roots reaching down into the earth. Repeat.

5. **Notice how this feels in your body.** Consider the type of tree you have imagined and name it. Your body will remember this feeling and the name. Take a moment to give thanks for giving yourself this experience, and when you are ready slowly blink your eyes open and take a few steps forward. Notice how your feet, legs, and body feel. Notice the strength and grounding in your body.

With practice, you can invoke the grounded feeling by recalling your tree and breathing.

CREATIVE PRACTICE 8:
Getting in touch with your breathing

Start the practice by assuming this posture:

+ Sit relaxed, spine straight, shoulders back, down and loose, with your hands on the arms of a chair or in your lap, not crossed, and your feet flat on the floor. You can also stand, feet shoulder-width apart and knees slightly bent, or lie down, flat on your back.

+ Place one hand on chest and one on your upper abdomen, above your navel.

+ Close your eyes to heighten the awareness of how you breathe. Do you breathe into your chest or into your abdomen? Do you breathe quickly, slowly, or at a moderate rate? Do you breathe through your nose or through your mouth? Find your own rhythm, then slow it down, just a little bit, with each breath.

Try these steps:

✦ With eyes closed, breathe through your nose, feeling the air move down into your lungs as your chest and belly slowly rise and your shoulders straighten.

✦ Exhale slowly through your mouth, and feel your abdomen and then your chest deflate and your shoulders relax.

✦ Continue breathing this way for 10 more breaths.

✦ Concentrate. Notice the slight temperature change between cool air entering your nose and warmer breath leaving your mouth. Follow your breath and imagine that you are traveling with it through your nose, nostrils, and swirling down into your lungs, then slowly pushing back out through your mouth.

✦ Right now know that all you have to do is breathe, nothing else. If your mind starts to wander, as it will, gently bring your concentration back to focus on breathing. You may need to do this often and that's all right. It may have been a while since you slowed down enough to be aware of your breathing. This quieter sensation of slowing your body down may seem unfamiliar.

Finish with a cleansing breath

✦ Breathe in deeply through your nose to a slow count of four, then hold your breath for another slow count of four.

✦ Exhale slowly through your mouth for a count of four.

✦ Push out the last bits of air through your mouth, making puffing sounds.

Try this cleansing breathing at the end of your exercise. Do this at least three times. Exhaling through your mouth is a stronger detoxifying breath than exhaling through your nose.

CREATIVE PRACTICE 9:
Breathing to breeze through your day

Proper breathing awareness can be incorporated into your daily life in many ways. Here's one helpful practice.

Imagine a string holding you attached to the sky.

Do this at your desk, in your car, walking, reading, on the phone, to start your day, to end your day, or even in anticipation of a stressful experience. Do it before a meal, or at the start of a meeting, before a test or in class. Do it whenever you want to calm or refresh yourself.

Start by paying attention to the way you usually breathe. Is it quick and shallow? When practicing deep breathing, slow down if you begin to feel light headed. Your body may not be used to all the oxygen it's getting. Like anything new, breathing deeply takes practice and getting used to.

If deep breathing is new to you, practice it before you combine it with other exercises and activities. When you set aside time for breathing, do so before meals or at least two hours after a meal, use a well-ventilated room or go outdoors, and wear loose clothing. This will help you to get the most benefit from your deep breathing.

Try giving yourself gentle reminders to breathe deeply until it becomes a habit. Place sticky notes on cupboards or mirrors, or inspirational posters or artwork that remind you to breathe deeply and slowly.

CREATIVE PRACTICE 10:
Everyday breathing exercises

These three breathing exercises take just moments, but can have lasting benefits.

1. Rejuvenating wake-up breathing

✦ Sit comfortably in a relaxed position.

✦ Inhale to a slow count of six.

✦ Hold for one count.

✦ Exhale for a slow count of three.

✦ Find your own rhythm. Be sure to breathe in longer than you breathe out, thus feeding yourself oxygen. Repeat until you feel wide awake.

2. Breathing to induce sleep and deep relaxation

✦ Lie or sit in a relaxed position.

✦ Inhale for three counts.

✦ Hold for one count.

✦ Exhale for six counts.

✦ As you breathe out, permit yourself to become increasingly relaxed by releasing the tension slowly out of your body with the exhaling breath. Repeat until you are relaxed or asleep.

3. Breathing to get in touch with yourself

✦ Just as breathing can relax and invigorate our bodies, so too can it relax and invigorate our minds. That's why the practice of meditation begins with awareness of our breathing.

CREATIVE PRACTICE 11:
Moving breathing (qigong)

Why moving? In moving I am more in my body and less in my head. Sometimes I need to move to slow down.

To help his warriors increase their attention and focus, Marshall Yueh Fei of the Sung Dynasty used a series of moving breathing exercises drawn from qigong, an ancient Chinese health care system that combines posture, breathing techniques, and focused intention.

Follow the steps of this particular breathing exercise and enjoy stretching your arms and expanding your lungs.

1. Stand looking straight ahead, with your feet shoulder-width apart, your back straight in the pelvic tilt position, and your knees slightly bent. (To assume a pelvic tilt position, pretend you are about to sit. As you begin to sit, your pelvis will slightly rock forward, your buttocks will sink slightly, and your balance will rest in the centre of your body.)

2. Gently intertwine your fingers and bring your arms out in front of you as if you are hugging a barrel. Lower your arms, keeping them around the imaginary barrel. With your arms in this position, breathe in, still hugging the barrel while slowly raising your arms to shoulder height. As you exhale gently, lower your arms slowly back to your navel.

3. Still in the hugging-the-barrel position, with fingers intertwined, breathe in and raise your arms above your head. Let your eyes follow your hands to the sky.

4. On the exhale, gently separate your fingers and gradually bring your arms down in a wide arc. Follow this motion in your peripheral vision until your arms reach shoulder height. Looking ahead, continue to bring your arms down to your belly as you finish exhaling.

When you breathe in, concentrate on expanding your lungs as much as you can. When you breathe out, concentrate on contracting your belly.

Steps one to four constitute one set. Depending on instructors and styles, there are many variations. Take your time to work up to six sets of this exercise.

CREATIVE PRACTICE 12:
Sitting breathing

✦ Assume the posture we used when first getting in touch with our breathing: sit relaxed, spine straight, shoulders back, down and loose, with your hands on the arms of a chair or in your lap, not crossed, and your feet flat on the floor.

✦   Sit alone in silence. Balance your head, close your eyes,
    breathe in and out gently, and imagine yourself looking
    into your heart.

✦   As you slow your breathing down a little, slow your
    thoughts down a little.

✦   Be calm, focusing solely on breathing.

✦   Slow your breathing a little more. Slow your thoughts a
    little more.

✦   If it's helpful, repeat a one-syllable word such as 'love' or
    'peace', or another word that fulfills you. Or, if you like,
    count each breath. For example, 'one' for the inhale,
    'two' for the exhale, 'three' for the next inhale, and so
    on. Focus on that word while leaving all other thoughts
    behind. Slow the word down a little at a time.

✦   Now try to imagine the space before and after that
    word. Focus on the spaces. This takes practice and
    concentration. In time, the spaces will get longer. When
    you can achieve this calm space, you will connect with
    the truth of energy and the universe. At this level, it is
    said that you will find your highest thoughts, and your
    wisdom will come to you.

CREATIVE PRACTICE 13:
Experiencing music in shapes and words

Here are three creative practices involving music.

Practice one

1. With your eyes closed, breathe deeply for a few minutes,
    and then listen attentively to a selected sound piece.

2. Let the shapes of the sounds drift into your mind.

3. With a pencil and paper, mark down the general line and/
    or shape that the particular sound prompts for you. For

example, a low note may appear large and round, and a high note may appear tight and small. Do the shapes feel connected or separate? When you are ready, continue with another piece.

Different rhythms in sounds may reflect your rhythm of transcribing; for example, for a fast beat, short, quick strokes. The sounds from different musical instruments will prompt various shapes and reactions.

Practice two

1. With a selection of crayons or markers in front of you, listen to a sound selection.

2. Breathe deeply and close your eyes. Open yourself to letting the music stimulate colour in your imagination. Record the shapes in colour as you listen to each musical piece. For example, a high note may appear bright for you.

3. To deepen your sound awareness and experience further, describe on a separate piece of paper the shapes and colours you just made. Use descriptors such as 'jagged, sharp line', 'round, thick lines', 'tiny, spiralling red lines', and so on. After you have done so, answer these questions:

   ✦ What did it feel like to paint from start to finish?

   ✦ Any distractions?

   ✦ What about the movement of the lines? Quick or slow?

I have shared this creative practice with different groups. We have numbered the pieces as we go along. In our sharing, it is fascinating to see that each musical piece had a character and feeling that we could collectively feel, along with our individual interpretations.

Practice three

This exercise takes the previous exercise a step further.

1. Listen to musical selections as suggested previously.

2. Write down or describe the thoughts, words, phrases, ideas, or memories that come to mind. Do not judge the process or order of your words. Just record them.

3. Any surprises? Have you discovered anything new?

4. Write as long as you wish.

5. How can you use these discoveries in your life?

The process of journaling accomplishes at least two important goals: It provides a reflective pause in your activities, and increasingly helps you to express yourself. It can be surprising what the journaling reveals, for instance, perhaps buried memories and/or glorious experiences. Perhaps you will learn new things about yourself. Sometimes you may organize the day, or the rest of your life and dreams. Other times, the journaling is just a way to clear one's mind.

CREATIVE PRACTICE 14:
Giving yourself to music

In dance, I can give myself to the rhythm of the music. I don't have to think or solve anything. My body can just physically be. Tap your toe, rock your head, sway, move any way you like. That's all. That's enough.

In this creative practice, first try experiencing the music in a space with no mirrors, so you do not feel any judgment on how you move, or if you move, or even how you look. Try this on your own or with a supportive group where it is safe to move without judgment or expectations.

Let yourself become one with the music. Imagine that you are swallowing the music and take it in deeply.

1. Try a song that you connect to. Try slow, soft songs, happy lyrical songs, hard, heavy songs, erratic, chaotic songs, and easy, smooth songs.

2. Sense your body. What are you feeling? How is your body responding? What areas react first? What parts of your body resist movement?

3. Try moving as if you are performing on a stage. Try moving as if you are with a lover.

4. Move as if you are in water. Remain acutely aware of your movements. Feel the energy of the music so you are not separate anymore. Become one with the music. Did you sweat? Did you have fun? Did you giggle or cry?

5. Sometimes while you are dancing, add your voice. Sing out loud! Yell! Moan! Sigh...

At the beginning, your voice might feel tight or shy. You have a wide range of tones and volumes. Use it all to express how you feel.

Notice how your voice can create different vibrations in your body.

Hum. Hum with the music and feel the vibrations of the humming inside yourself. Hum throughout the day, then note how you feel.

How would you draw your dance? How would you paint your dance? Be still...

What is happening in your body?

CREATIVE PRACTICE 15:
Journaling — emptying the clutter from your mind

From time to time, empty your mind of all those words tumbling about that may be giving you a headache or holding back an avalanche of creative possibilities.

This exercise will help you to loosen up your mind and relax the usual meticulousness of your thoughts and judgments. This practice is a warm-up to help clean out the brain's cobwebs and perhaps uncover a gem of a thought, or release an avalanche of creative possibilities.

1. Using a pad of paper, a scribbler, a loose-leaf binder or a blank bound book, just write whatever comes to mind. Be relaxed. Have fun. This creative practice is for your eyes only.

Pretend that you are the recording secretary for your thoughts. Edit nothing. Write whatever comes to mind, even if it is incomplete, even if your brain is rebelling, or you are thinking that you are stuck. Record it all. I tell my students it's all right to record a shopping list if that is what comes to mind, or even to write, "I feel awkward." As you write down those seemly idle words as they come to mind no matter what they are new words and thoughts will replace them.

2. Use a timer so that you are not preoccupied with looking at the time. Set it for 10 minutes. As you become accustomed to journaling, write for as long as you need to.

There is no pressure here to produce a product. This is just for you.

CREATIVE PRACTICE 16:
Gratitude Attitude

Pick a time of day when it's most convenient to journal briefly. Use a small notebook, or even strips of paper that you keep in a box or jar, to list in point form things for which you're grateful. It doesn't matter how big or small these things are, or if you're grateful for the same things day after day.

I gratitude journal in the morning and in the evening, and here are some of the things I write down:

+ waking up
+ my healthy body
+ my comfy bed
+ the new day, 84,000 seconds
+ my children
+ my pets

+ morning coffee
+ a phone
+ good dreams
+ faith
+ trust
+ and so on...

I liked how this made me feel, so I began writing a list in the evening too, before sleep. Because the journal was tiny it also could travel easily with me. I kept it up, and after a few months I noticed that I was waking up with a smile on my face and going to sleep with a smile on my face. I used to suffer from insomnia, now I sleep very solidly most nights. I like that. This practice has grown into a larger book and it is one of the most treasured times of day for me. It does not matter how I wake up; by the time I have finished my daily practice I am grounded and have chosen the channel of gratitude in my brain.

> It is not happy people who are grateful.
> It is people who are grateful that are happy.

CREATIVE PRACTICE 17:

Developing supportive tools

Start writing a simple list of the things that you enjoy, and that just make you feel good. Lists are good to have handy—they are especially supportive when we are tired . . . too weary to think clearly to the next step. Turning to such tools when times are tough or when you are feeling low or insecure can help to renew your energy and lift your mood.

The following is part of my support list. Create your own list under these headings:

Spiritual
- Meditation
- Chanting
- Singing
- Reading
- Support group
- Long walks
- Deep breathing

Mental
- Study
- Movies
- Books

Physical
- Bike riding
- Skiing
- Dancing
- Camping

Sensual
- Fresh air
- Sunshine
- Lovely clothes
- Time with my lover
- Slow dancing

Emotional
- Playing with my children
- Hugs
- A puppy

Set up a blank chart with the above headings on a separate page. There is no right or wrong for where things are placed. Some activities overlap in various categories.

CREATIVE PRACTICE 18:

Supportive chart

I designed this chart to include things I regularly do, as well as things I want more support on. Occasionally, I modify the chart.

The more checks I have, the better I feel. Awarding myself check marks helps me to include more positive things in my life, and even to trim off a few pounds. For each chart I complete, I give myself a reward.

Whenever I find myself getting worn down and tired or feeling overwhelmed, then I know it's time to pull out this chart. It quickly lets me know what I've been neglecting. Below is my own example, but you can create your own categories.

Every day, 'feed' all aspects of yourself, including your spiritual, emotional, mental, physical and sensual aspects.

SUPPORTIVE CHART															
Morning stretch															
Breathing															
Journal writing															
Gratitude list															
A walk															
Other exercise															
Taking a rest															
Spiritual reading															
Humming, singing															
Sunshine															
Hugs															
Fun															
Healthy snacks, apples															
More veggies															
Evening stretch															

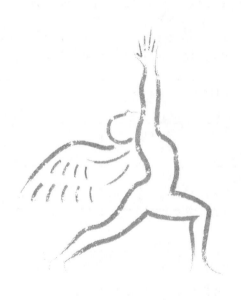

Your Own Anxiety Warrior

If I could only give you two words from this book, they would be *awareness* and *practice*.

Become aware so you know what to change/ modify/manage and practice in your strategies.

Life is a process and a practice for all of us!

No matter what type of anxiety you're dealing with, anxiety can be managed by the following strategies:

✦ Explore and understand the possibility of a specific type of anxiety.

✦ Accept your anxiety as a gift, a signal, an opportunity, a message.

✦ Identify and understand the causes and triggers for your anxiety.

✦ Use the scale 0 to 10 to identify the intensity of your anxiety.

✦ Know your limits (sleep, hunger, amount and type of stressors).

✦ Perhaps break down your anxiety into smaller layers.

✦ Manage the easy layers first, right away.

✦ Change your lifestyle to lower your anxiety.

✦   Practice your strategies.

✦   Create your own daily practice and practice it daily,
     especially when you feel pleasant.

As you have read, there are many facets to anxiety. It is more than
just a word or condition. Anxiety can be a gift, an opportunity inviting us to look deeper into ourselves. I hope that you have found inspiration to explore and sooth those tender parts of yourself.

I used to curse anxiety and its symptoms. I hated it! I tried to tame
it, chase it away with a stick or a song. I thought it was weak and sick.
When I began to be curious, and I cautiously ventured closer to it, to
try and understand it. As I explored anxiety, it showed me myself and
my life. I learned about the vulnerable part of me, that was worthy of
love and kindness and of thriving. I hope this book has gently opened
some doors for your curiosity. You are worth it! We can do this!

Glossary

ANXIETY: state of worry, nervousness, or unease, typically about an imminent event or something with an uncertain outcome. Feeling; concern, apprehension, unease, fearful, disquiet, agitation, angst, tension, twitchiness, nervousness. Mostly felt in anticipation of something happening. It is a natural alarm response that helps people to avoid dangerous situations and is a signal to motivate them to solve everyday problems.

ANXIETY DISORDER: Anxiety disorders are mental health problems characterized by excessive levels of alarm, fear or worry due to anticipated or perceived danger. They significantly interfere with day-to-day living. There are many different types of anxiety disorders, including bipolar disorder and depressive disorder (depression).

BELIEFS: Beliefs are firm opinions or convictions. Belief systems are a set of beliefs or principles that characterize a community, religion, or philosophy. They are often influenced by culture, which in turn guides behaviour and communication. Cultural belief systems can shape a person's understanding of health and illness.

BIPOLAR DISORDER: Bipolar disorder is a type of mood disorder in which a person alternates between states of clinical depression and mania. Bipolar disorder is sometimes called manic depression.

COMMUNITY MENTAL HEALTH TEAM (CMHT): CMHTs look after the welfare of people who need more attention to their mental health problems than a family doctor can provide. Care teams vary from area to area and can include psychiatrists, psychologists, community psychiatric nurses, social workers, housing and welfare officers.

DELUSIONS: Delusions are fixed, false beliefs that are not culturally sanctioned. They may arise from distorted interpretations of reality. They may include beliefs of persecution, guilt, having a special mission or being under outside control. No matter how bizarre the delusions may seem to others, the people experiencing them believe they are real.

DEPRESSIVE DISORDER (DEPRESSION): Depression is characterized by either a sad or irritable mood, or the loss of interest or enjoyment in nearly all activities for a period of at least two weeks. Depression is more than short-term feelings of sadness.

EMDR: This stands for Eye Movement Desensitization and Reprocessing, though it does not have much to do with the eyes. This therapy uses bi-lateral movement stimulation in which eyes move back and forth, or bi-lateral body movement, like tapping or wearing a headset using alternating beeps or music.

EMDR was developed in the late 80s in the US and was primarily used for war veterans with PTSD. It has quickly come to be useful in eliminating all the symptoms associated with stress and trauma, like flashbacks, panic attacks, intrusive thoughts, anxiety, phobias, depression, over-reactive anger, worrying, disturbed sleep, and so on. It has been studied and validated all around the world.

Sometimes, memories get stuck in the information processing system of the brain, along with pictures, sounds, smells, tastes, emotions, and body sensations, which were all part of the original experience. When memories are stuck, this is where EMDR, 'desensitizes and reprocesses' the memory, helping the brain reprocess the memory, to a point where remembering the event no longer bothers you and you have peace with it.

Science does not know exactly how the brain files the memories during EMDR. It is similar to the dream stage, or Rapid Eye Movement (REM) stage of sleep. EMDR may be a kind of accelerated, conscious version of REM sleep.

EMDR is approved as an evidence-based, best-practice trauma therapy for PTSD and related issues by many international health and government bodies, including the World Health

Organization (WHO) in 2013, the American Psychological Association (APA) in 2004 and 2009, and the American Department of Defense/Veterans' Affairs (2004 and 2010).

FEAR: Fear happens when something threatens you, while worry is being afraid in anticipation of something happening. They both have the same physiological response in the body. Fear is when you are in the woods and a bear is coming after you. You must make a decision, you are afraid, you must run or take cover. Fear is an important human emotion. It has kept us alive as a human race.

MANIA: Mania is one of the emotional extremes associated with bipolar disorder. Mania is characterized by an elevated mood, grandiose ideas, and irritability for a period of at least one week. The start is usually sudden and can increase rapidly over a few days.

MASLOW'S HIERARCHY: Maslow's hierarchy of needs is usually depicted like this triangle: In 1943, American psychologist Abraham Maslow was curious about what motivated humans. He surmised that the most basic physiological needs for survival were the most important, such as air, shelter, warmth, water, food, and rest. It is important to feel secure and safe, to have protection from the elements, and a sense of stability. These are the most fundamental and crucial needs. As shown in the illustration, love and belonging and self esteem are also considered basic needs.

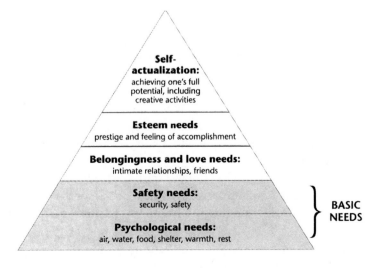

His theory was that when humans had their basic needs met, then they could progress to higher goals such as self-actualization, self-fulfillment and achievement. His research showed that as the quality of their needs rose so did the quality of their activities, production and creativity.

In the event that humans needed to struggle to meet basic needs of survival, or in the event these needs were not met, humans would experience stress, tension, uncertainty, fear, and anxiety.

MENTAL DISORDER: A mental disorder causes major changes in a person's thinking, emotional state and behaviour, and disrupts the person's ability to work and carry out their usual personal relationships.

MENTAL HEALTH: Mental health is a state of well-being in which individuals realize their own abilities, can cope with the normal stresses of life, can work productively, and are able to make a contribution to their community.

MENTAL HEALTH PROBLEM: A mental health problem is a broad term that includes both mental disorders and symptoms that may not be severe enough to warrant the diagnosis of a mental disorder.

MOOD DISORDER: Mood disorders are mental health problems characterized by disturbances in the way a person feels and experiences emotion, and which make it difficult for the person to function in day-to-day life.

PATHOLOGICAL ANXIETY: Psychiatric meaning; a nervous disorder characterized by a state of excessive uneasiness and apprehension, typically with compulsive behaviour or panic attacks. When anxiety is a problem it affects our health, our well-being, our happiness and health. When anxiety stops us from doing something, like going out of the house, going shopping, driving, taking a course, going to a party, or visiting family, it is a problem.

PSYCHIATRIST: Psychiatrists are medical doctors who specialize in mental health and mental illness. Psychiatrists make diagnoses, decisions about treatment and care, and prescribe psychiatric drugs and therapies.

PSYCHOLOGIST: Psychologists study the human mind and its effects on behaviour. Psychologists can use behaviour therapy to help people work through the way they act in certain situations.

SELF-ESTEEM: Self-esteem is the way we feel about ourselves and our abilities and reflects the value we place on ourselves as human beings.

SELF-STIGMA: The prejudice and discrimination people face because of mental health problems often become internalized. People with mental health problems begin to believe the negative things that other people and the media say about them. They have lower self-esteem because they feel guilt and shame. As a result, they often do not seek the help they need.

STIGMA: Stigma refers to negative attitudes (prejudices) and negative behaviours (discrimination) toward people with substance use and mental health problems. Stigma means having fixed ideas and judgments about people as well as feeling disgust and avoiding what we don't understand. Stigma results in the exclusion of people with mental health problems from activities that are open to other people such as getting a job, finding a safe place to live, participating in social activities and having relationships.

STIMULANTS: Caffeine has a directly stimulating effect on several different systems in the body. Too much caffeine can keep you in a tense, aroused condition, leaving you more vulnerable to generalized anxiety as well as panic attacks. For those people who are very sensitive to caffeine, less than 50 mg/day is advisable.

STIMULANTS: Nicotine is as strong a stimulant as caffeine. It stimulates increased physiological arousal and makes the heart work harder. People who smoke are more prone to anxiety states and panic.

STRESS: Stress is a demand on physical or mental energy that may or may not disturb a person's normal functioning.

References

A Course in Miracles. The Foundation for Inner Peace, Viking, New York, NY, 1996. *(A non-denominational book on God, Jesus and Living. A very heavy book, best studied with groups.)*

Allen, James. *As a Man Thinketh.* Thomas Y. Crowell Co., New York, NY, 1902.

Attwood, Janet, and Chris Attwood, *The Passion Test, The Effortless Path to Discovering Your Life Purpose,* Penguin Books, New York, NY, 2007.

Balch, Phyllis, A, CNC, Prescription for Nutritional Healing, Avery, New York NY, 2000. *(This book is updated regularly, watch for the newest edition.)*

Bassett, Lucinda. *From Panic to Power,* HarperCollins, New York, NY, 1997. *(Easy to read; the author uses many of her personal experiences in a humorous way. Included are many support points for anxiety and worry.)*

Benson, Herbert. *The Relaxation Response.* William Morrow and Company, New York, NY, 1975.

Bourne, Edmund PhD, *The Anxiety and Phobia Workbook,* New Harbinger Publications, Oakland, CA, 2015.

Bilodeau, Lorraine. *The Anger Workbook.* Hazelden Foundation, Center City, MN, 1994. *(A simple workbook designed to get you thinking, understanding, and redirecting your frustration and angry feelings.)*

Brown, Brené. *The Gifts of Imperfection.* Hazelden Publishing, Center City, MN, 2010.

Buettner, Dan. *The Blue Zones,* Lessons for living longer from the people who've lived the longest. National Geographic, Washington, DC, 2008.

Cameron, Julia. *The Artist's Way.* Tarcher/Perigee, New York, NY, 1992. *(A 12-week program to help readers discover their creative self and their creative blocks. Lots of applications; best done with a buddy or in a group.)*

Campbell, Don. *The Mozart Effect.* Avon Books, The Hearst Corporation, New York, NY, 1997.

Canfield, Jack. *The Success Principles.* HarperCollins, New York, NY, 2007.

Chancellor, Philip M., *Illustrated Handbook of the Bach Flowers Remedies.* Hillman Printers, Great Britain, 1971.

Dennison, Paul E., and Gail E. Dennison. *Brain Gym.* Edu-Kinesthetics, Ventura, CA, 1986. *(Many practical exercises to relax, rejuvenate, and stimulatebrainactivity.)*

Dispenza, Joe. *You Are the Placebo.* Hay House, Carlsbad, CA, 2014. *(This book is about you making your mind matter in creating your health and your life. It is backed by science and a team of doctors.)*

Ikeda, Daisaku. *Faith into Action.* World Tribune Press, Santa Monica, CA, 1999. *(A collection containing reflections for many life situations. Based on a Buddhist perspective.)*

Doidage, Norman, *The Brain that Changes Itself,* Penguin Books, New York, NY, 2007.

Franck, Frederick. *The Zen of Seeing,* Random House, New York, NY, 1973.

Frankl, Victor, *Man's Search for Meaning,* Washington Square Press, New York, NY, 1984.

Gawain, Shakti. *Creative Visualization: Meditations.* New World Library, Novato, CA, 1995.

Gendlin, Eugene T. *Focusing,* Bantam Books, New York, NY, 1978 and 1982.

Goldberg, Natalie. *Writing Down the Bones.* Shambhala Press, Boston, MA, 1986. *(All her books are excellent guides to stimulate the writer in you. Another way to self-discovery through writing.)*

Goldstein, Nathan. *The Art of Responsive Drawing.* Prentice Hall, Upper Saddle River, NJ, 1973.

Goleman, David. *Emotional Intelligence.* Bantam Books, New York, NY, 1995.

Gray, John. *Practical Miracles for Mars and Venus.* HarperCollins, New York, NY, 1999.

Hart, Mickey with Jay Stevens. *Drumming at the Edge of Magic.* Harper Colling, San Francisco, CA, 1960.

Hay, Louise. *You Can Heal Your Life*. Hay House, Carlsbad, CA, 1999.

Heath, Yvonne, *Love Your Life to Death: How to Plan and Prepare for End of Life so You Can Live Fully Now*. Port Sydney, ON, 2015

Jenkinson, Stephen, *How It Could All Be: A work book for dying people and for those that love them*, First Choice Books, Victoria, BC, 2009.

Jeffers, Sue, Dr., *Feel the Fear and Do It Anyway*. Random House, London, UK, 1991.

Kavelin Popov, Linda. *The Family Virtues Guide*. Plume Books, Penguin Group, New York, NY, 1997. (*A basic book about morals and character.*)

Kriz, Jurgen, *Self Actualization*, Germany, Books on Demand, 2006.

Liedloff, Jean. *The Continuum Concept*. Addison-Wesley Publication Co. Inc., Reading, MA, 1985.

May, Rollo. *The Courage to Create*. Norton, New York, NY, 1975.

Murdock, Maureen. *Spinning Inward: guided imagery for children for learning, creativity and relaxation*. Shambala Publications, Boston, MA, 1987.

Nicolaides, Kimon. *The Natural Way to Draw*. Houghton Mifflin Company, Boston, MA, 1969.

Pearson, Carol. *The Hero Within*. HarperCollins, New York, NY, 1991. (*Various human characteristics illustrated using hero characters.*)

Peck, M. Scott. *The Road Less Travelled*. Simon & Schuster, New York, NY, 1978.

Pitman, Walter, Ontario Arts Council. *Making the Case for Arts Education*. Ontario Arts Council, Toronto, ON, 1997.

Pearce, Joseph. *Magical Child*. Penguin Group, New York, NY, 1997.

Rinpoche, Sogyal. *The Tibetan Book of Living and Dying*. HarperOne, San Francisco, CA, 2002.

Rosenberg, Marshall. *The Surprising Purpose of Anger. Beyond Anger Management: Finding the Gift*. PuddleDancer Press,. (*Rosenberg won 11 peace awards for his work,* Nonviolent Communication: A Language of Life. *There are many YouTube videos online and he has many small books explaining his model.*)

Roth, Gabrielle. *Maps to Ecstasy: Teachings of an Urban Shaman*. New World Library, San Rafael, CA, 1989.

Shinn, Florence, *Your Word Is Your Wand,* Essex, UK, Dotesios Printers Ltd., Essex, UK, 1928.

Shinn, Florence, *The Game of Life,* Essex, UK, Dotesios Dotesios Printers Ltd., 1928.

Sobel, Elliot. *Wild Heart Dancing*. Fireside Press, New York, NY, 1987. (*A self-directed private creativity retreat. To be taken along and only read as you complete exercises. Lots of fun and worthwhile*).

Tavris, Carol. *Anger: the Misunderstood Emotion*. Simon&Schuster, New York, NY, 1982.

Tisserand, Robert B., *The Art of Aromatherapy*, Destiny Books, Rochester, VL, 1977.

Tolle, Eckhart, *Power of Now*, Namaste Publishing, Vancouver, BC, 1997.

Tolle, Eckhart, *A New Earth, Awakening to your Life's Purpose*, Plume, Penguin Group, New York, NY, 2006.

Von Oech, Roger. *A Whack on the Side of the Head*. Warner Books, New York, NY, 1998.

Zukav, Gary, *The Seat of the Soul*. Shambhala Publications, Boston, MA, 1991.

About the Contributors

Ryan Brown

Ryan Brown specializes in debt management and financial restructuring. He has been assisting Canadians at becoming debt free since 2010 by operating three 4 Pillars Consulting Group offices in Ontario: Muskoka and Parry Sound; Sudbury; and North Bay. With locations across the country, 4 Pillars consultants like Ryan offer a variety of services specific to people in debt.

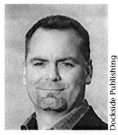

Among Ryan's clients, less than one 1% file bankruptcy. Many become debt free within 24 to 36 months. With a passion for his work and belief in the solutions 4 Pillars offers, Ryan is motivated to publicly address complex financial issues, such as Canada's highly leveraged banking system, the devaluation of currency versus inflation, Canadian household and business debt challenges, insolvency options, and corresponding topics. Ryan is often heard saying that, in some capacity, he will likely be in this line of work for the rest of his life. Contact Ryan at 705-640-0187; www.4pillars.ca/on/muskoka and sudburydebtfree.ca.

Julie Bissonette

Julie Bissonette is a consultant with Investors Group Financial Services Inc. and she has lived in Bracebridge, Ontario since 1988. She prides herself on her strong customer service skills and her genuine interest in helping those in her community. Since 2013, Julie has been assisting her clients by composing financial plans to ensure their future is secure and helping them achieve

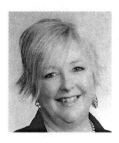

their most important financial goals. Julie is often quoted as saying that "This is the best career I've ever had as I love helping people and seeing them reach their goals. At Investors Group, our vision is to improve our clients' financial well-being...and I get to help my clients do this every day." Julie plans to continue her career with Investors Group for many more years. julie.bissonette@investorsgroup.com

The views of Julie Bissonette in this publication are those of the author. Julie Bissonette is responsible for the content she provided to this publication. Investors Group Financial Services Inc. or Investors Group Securities Inc. and its affiliates are not responsible for and cannot accept any liability for any information in this publication.

Yvonne Heath

Married to her best friend Geordie and mother of three, Yvonne Heath lives in beautiful Muskoka.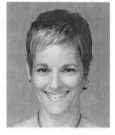

During 27 years of nursing she witnessed society's death phobia and how our reluctance to talk about, plan, and prepare for grief, death and dying causes excessive suffering. She suffered too. At age 50 she left her career and blazed a new trail.

Her new purpose is to empower compassionate communities and professionals to live life to the fullest, to learn to grieve and support others, and to have 'The Talk' about end of life long before people have to face it. To share her message, she has written a book entitled *Love Your Life to Death*, become an Inspirational speaker, a TV host, and author of a website, blog and Facebook page.

Read more about Yvonne Heath and her book on her website: www.loveyourlifetodeath.com.

Jill Hewlett

As a nationally recognized Wellness Authority, Brain Fitness Expert, and Brain Gym consultant for two decades, Jill Hewlett has the skillful capacity to draw out the natural leadership and vitality in individuals of all ages, as well as community groups and organizations, and to support them in reducing stress and achieving greater levels of efficiency, mental health, work/ life balance, and success.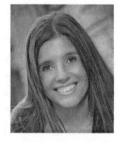

Jill is the founder of the Women's Wellness Circles. She began her first circle over a decade ago. Today they continue to grow and expand into the many locations that she mentors. These circles nourish, educate and inspire women in their communities.

Author of *Common Sense, Uncommonly Practised: A Heartfelt Book about Achieving Personal Wellness*, Jill has a passion and talent for making life changes and improvements easy and attainable for all those who want it. www.jillhewlett.com.

Bari McFarland

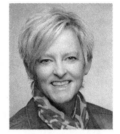

Author, speaker and certified life coach, Bari works with clients worldwide who know there is something more to life and just don't know how to get there. With over 25 years of experience applying the tools and techniques for positive living, Bari offers personalized coaching, as well as retreats and corporate workshops that help clients create the life and reality they want.

Whether you are feeling unfulfilled in your current career, in business or in life, or are in transition, Bari is here to help you uncover to recover, and enhance your quality of life through self-discovery, self-empowerment and creating the habits necessary to make your ideal life a reality.

Visit www.mydharma.ca to explore the exciting retreats and workshops Bari offers. Book her for a speaking engagement or corporate event, and register for her popular daily affirmations. She'd also love to connect with you on Facebook (www.facebook.com/MyDharma-FanPage) and Twitter @bariccp.

Suzanne Witt-Foley

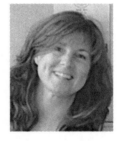

Suzanne Witt-Foley is a dynamic and experienced speaker and educator. She has created and delivered hundreds of presentations nationally. Passionate to build understanding about mental health and addiction, she engages her audience by exploring our fast paced, toxically stressed culture and why now, more than ever, building relationships and community connectedness is essential to our well-being.

As an innovator in knowledge exchange, training and education, Suzanne has over 25 years of experience in community development and capacity building.

Suzanne was employed as a community consultant for the Centre for Addiction and Mental Health (CAMH) for over 16 years and has worked in a variety of other settings in Ontario and Eastern Canada. Suzanne is currently one of Ontario's leading Mental Health First Aid Instructors and has provided 50 Mental Health First Aid training events since January 2014. She has certified over 800 participants and has received glowing reviews. Learn more about Suzanne's work at www.suzannewittfoley.com.

About the Author

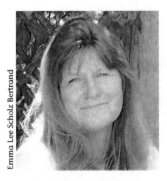

Emma Lee Scholz Bertrand

Elke Scholz, MA, RP, REACE, is a well-known author, therapist, speaker, and facilitator. She was awarded a Masters degree in Expressive Arts Therapy by European Graduate School (EGS), Saas Fee, Switzerland. She is internationally certified in EMDR and is a registered expressive arts consultant/educator (REACE) with the International Expressive Arts Therapy Association (IEATA).

All her life, Elke has understood the connection between the arts and living. For her, the elements connect at every level, and she is able to simplify concepts and relay this to other people in a simple, approachable way. Elke communicates this understanding, as well as her own artistic vision, in numerous ways.

Elke has been helping people since 1980. Her calm approach invites a comfortable space for people to try new things. Elke can be with clients in their darkest, hardest times. Her acute awareness and high sensitivity are tremendous assets for her clients and make her distinctive in her field. Elke works well with teams of educators, social workers, doctors, corporations, organizations, and groups. Other facilitators immensely enjoy her training sessions.

Programs for Youth

Most of Elke's program development work focuses on attachment, grief, trauma, and loss recovery using Expressive Arts. She successfully manages her own anxiety and gladly shares her success strategies. Elke's focus is on building the strengths of young people. She facilitates youth grief and loss recovery programs that she designed and developed for a regional hospice in Muskoka, Ontario.

Other group programs, which she facilitates in schools, are successful in assisting youth-at-risk with creative living and learning to become re-engaged with life, with attending class, and gaining life skills.

Frame of Reference

+ Curiosity
+ Mystery
+ Discovery
+ Guidance
+ Leadership
+ Non-positional, flexible, client-centred solutions

Elke's Own Creative Daily Principles and Practices

+ Daily gratitude journaling, morning and evening.
+ Long meditative walks through nature.
+ Joyfully hand-raising chickens, as egg layers, therapy aids, and entertainment.
+ Writing poetry.
+ Community drumming workshops.
+ Learning to play the flute and the piano.
+ Hiking, mountain biking, kayaking, and sketching in the great, wondrous outdoors.
+ Inspirational reading.
+ Exploring philosophy and spirituality with different local discussion groups.
+ Exploring life, love, and the universe.
+ Expressing it all in painting and sketches.

Please write to the publisher to let Elke know how this book works for you, or what you would like to see added to future editions.

The Artist's Reply

1060 Partridge Lane, Bracebridge, ON P1L 1W8
Tel: 705-646-2300
Email: elkescholz@theartistsreply.com

Visit www.elkescholz.com:
Free downloads, posters, radio talks, YouTube videos,
and many more resources.

To book Elke for speaking engagements and workshops:
Tel: 705.646.2300
Email: elkescholz@theartistsreply.com

Available in print and ebook format online or inquire at your local bookstore

ORDER MORE COPIES

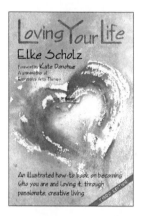

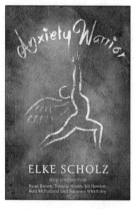

Loving Your Life, 3rd ed.

The third addition of this award-winning book with a foreword by Kate Donohue, a grandmother of EXA. Explore your creative mindfulness in this expressive arts book. Use it for daily inspirations, creative exercises and practices, for personal use, and in workshops. It is a fun and refreshing practical approach for well-being and for coming back to who you are.

Anxiety Warrior

This practical resource book is full of strategies and skills to manage and overcome anxiety. This book would have saved me a lot of pain if I'd had it in the past. Along with myself, there are five contributors. They are published authors, key note speakers, leaders and they are all professionals who are passionate about their work and empowering people

---

Also available from The Artist's Reply

1060 Partridge Lane, Bracebridge, ON P1L 1W8
Tel: 705-646-2300   elkescholz@theartistsreply.com

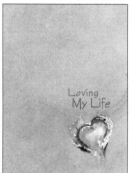

"Loving My Life" Journal

Journaling is a valuable activity that changes the neural pathways in our brain. Writing "it" down is a way to lessening our burdens. There is much research backing up the benefits of journaling. This journal provides 27 ideas to help initiate some personal exploration. Try, explore and play. Discover the ones you like and the ones that give you the most energy.